Melvin Delgado, PhD

Social Services in Latino Communities
Research and Strategies

*Pre-publication
REVIEWS,
COMMENTARIES,
EVALUATIONS . . .*

"**T**he clarity and definitiveness with which Delgado discusses practice with this specific community enhances practitioner knowledge by providing a perspective and strategies for informed practice with other Latino communities in the United States. . . . Sharpens intellectual understanding and practice implications for understanding and working with natural support systems."

Betty Garcia, PhD, MSW
Associate Professor,
Department of Social Work Education,
California State University, Fresno

"**D**emonstrates a keen knowledge and awareness of the dynamics of providing social work services to Latino communities. The book goes far beyond superficial cultural awareness and the traditional problem-focused method and presents a clearly developed strengths approach to social work practice. . . . Identifies community and cultural assets that are valuable tools when working with Latinos. . . . Delgado models empowerment by using youth and elderly community members as key informants and interviewees to identify assets in the community."

Juan Paz, DSW
Associate Professor,
School of Social Work,
Arizona State University

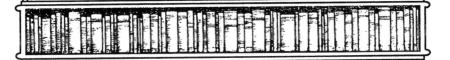

Social Services in Latino Communities
Research and Strategies

THE HAWORTH PRESS
New, Recent, and Forthcoming Titles
of Related Interest

Social Work Practice: A Systems Approach by Benyamin Chetkow-Yanoov

Elements of the Helping Process: A Guide for Clinicians by Raymond Fox

Clinical Social Work Supervision, Second Edition by Carlton E. Munson

Intervention Research: Design and Development for the Human Services edited by Jack Rothman and Edwin J. Thomas

Forensic Social Work: Legal Aspects of Professional Practice by Robert L. Barker and Douglas M. Branson

Now Dare Everything: Tales of HIV-Related Psychotherapy by Steven F. Dansky

The Black Elderly: Satisfaction and Quality of Later Life by Marguerite M. Coke and James A. Twaite

Building on Women's Strengths: A Social Work Agenda for the Twenty-First Century by Liane V. Davis

Family Beyond Family: The Surrogate Parent in Schools and Other Community Agencies by Sanford Weinstein

The Cross-Cultural Practice of Clinical Case Management in Mental Health edited by Peter Manoleas

Environmental Practice in the Human Services: Integration of Micro and Macro Roles, Skills, and Contexts by Bernard Neugeboren

Basic Social Policy and Planning: Strategies and Practice Methods by Hobart A. Burch

Fundamentals of Cognitive-Behavior Therapy: From Both Sides of the Desk by Bill Borcherdt

Social Work Intervention in an Economic Crisis: The River Communities Project by Martha Baum and Pamela Twiss

The Relational Systems Model for Family Therapy: Living in the Four Realities by Donald R. Bardill

Feminist Theories and Social Work: Approaches and Applications by Christine Flynn Saulnier

Social Work Approaches to Conflict Resolution: Making Fighting Obsolete by Benyamin Chetkow-Yanoov

Principles of Social Work Practice: A Generic Practice Approach by Molly R. Hancock

Nobody's Children: Orphans of the HIV Epidemic by Steven F. Dansky

Social Work in Health Settings: Practice in Context, Second Edition by Toba Schwaber Kerson and Associates

Critical Social Welfare Issues: Tools for Social Work and Health Care Professionals edited by Arthur J. Katz, Abraham Lurie, and Carlos Vidal

Social Work Practice: A Systems Approach, Second Edition by Benyamin Chetkow-Yanoov

Social Services in Latino Communities: Research and Strategies by Melvin Delgado

Social Services in Latino Communities
Research and Strategies

Melvin Delgado, PhD

The Haworth Press
New York • London

The Haworth Press, Inc., 10 Alice Street, Binghamton, NY 13904-1580

Cover design by Marylouise E. Doyle.

Library of Congress Cataloging-in-Publication Data

Delgado, Melvin.
    Social services in Latino communities : research and strategies / Melvin Delgado.
        p.   cm.
    Includes bibliographical references (p.   ) and index.
    ISBN 0-7890-0429-1 (alk. paper)
    1. Hispanic Americans—Services for. 2. Hispanic Americans—Services for—New England. 3. Puerto Ricans—Services for—United States. 4. Puerto Ricans—Services for—New England. 5. Social service—United States. 6. Social service—New England. I. Title.
HV3187.A2D44 1998
362.84′68073—DC21

                                                                            97-28881
                                                                            CIP

CONTENTS

ABOUT THE AUTHOR

Melvin Delgado, PhD, is Professor and Chair of Macro-Practice Sequence in the School of Social Work at Boston University. A faculty member there since 1979, he has also served the university as the Acting Coordinator of the Racism-Oppression Sequence and as Chairperson of the Community Organization, Management, and Planning Sequence. He has been principal investigator on many studies funded by organizations such as the Center on Substance Abuse Prevention, the Carlisle Foundation, the Massachusetts Department of Education, the U.S. Department of Education, and the National Institutes of Health. In 1994, he received the award for the Greatest Contribution to Social Work Education from the National Association of Social Work, Massachusetts Chapter, and in 1996, he received the Outstanding Contribution to the Boston University School of Social Work Alumni Award. A member of the Editorial Board of the *Journal of Multicultural Social Work, Social Work with Groups,* and *Alcoholism Treatment Quarterly,* Professor Delgado is co-editor of the book *Social Work Approaches to Alcohol and Other Drug Problems: Case Studies and Teaching Tools for Educators and Practitioners* and is the author of *Social Work Practice in Non-Traditional Urban Settings* (in press, Oxford University Press). He is also the author or co-author of numerous government reports, book chapters, and articles that have appeared in such journals as *Health and Social Work, Social Work in Education, Drugs & Society,* and *Social Work.*

Introduction

The Latino community in the United States presents the field of human services with a wide range of rewards and challenges. This population group is increasing numerically, is highly diverse in composition, and is dispersed throughout the United States, with major urban areas having a disproportionately large number of Latinos (Frisbie and Bean, 1995; Hurtado, 1995; Ortiz, 1995). Latinos, according to the 1990 U.S. Census Bureau, numbered approximately 27 million, with Mexican Americans (17 million), Puerto Ricans (2.8 million), and Cubans (1.1 million) as the three largest subgroups (IPR Datanote, 1995). However, there were approximately 3.7 million Central and South Americans and close to 2 million other Latinos (IPR Datanote, 1995). Latinos are expected to continue to increase numerically and number 51 million by 2020 and 81 million by 2050, making them the largest ethnic group in the United States (Pear, 1992; *The New York Times*, 1994).

The current and projected numbers, along with the unique challenges that these groups present for culturally competent research and service delivery, warrant a closer examination of the issues that must be successfully addressed by human service agencies and providers. These issues transcend a number of key factors: (1) the initiation of research that is centered on the circumstances and context in which Latinos live and function, and takes into account differences within and between groups; (2) the importance of agencies increasing their staff by hiring and supporting (supervision and training) bilingual and bicultural professionals who are Latino; (3) the need to develop innovative models of service delivery based upon assets rather than deficit paradigms; and (4) the assessment of the role of natural support systems within communities, and development of strategies for engaging these resources in collaboration partnerships.

This book consists of seven chapters published in the last few years based upon the author's research, consultation, and delivery of services to Puerto Ricans and other Latino groups in the United States. Much of the work in this book, however, focuses on the New England region, Massachusetts in particular. However, two of the articles take a more national perspective on the topic of Latinos with attention paid to Cubans, Mexican Americans, and Puerto Ricans. The approaches and issues raised throughout this book, nevertheless, have implications for other sections of the United States and Latino groups other than Puerto Ricans.

This book is divided into two sections. The first section focuses on research and the second on developing approaches to outreaching, engaging, and serving Latinos. The chapter titled "Community Asset Assessment and Substance Abuse Prevention: A Case Study Involving the Puerto Rican Community" provides the readers with a paradigm and methodology for addressing a community's assets rather than needs. This chapter describes in detail the process for planning and implementing an assessment of indigenous resources by utilizing residents as interviewers. The following chapter ("Puerto Rican Elders and Gerontological Research: Avenues for Empowerment and Participation") examines research with elders that utilizes an empowerment paradigm, and explores a variety of ways for engaging Latinos in undertaking research within their own communities. The chapter, although focused on elders, has implications for other age groups.

The second section of the book consists of five chapters focused on various aspects of service delivery to Puerto Ricans and other Latinos. Religion is often mentioned as playing a very important role in the lives of Latino elders and other age groups. Chapter 3, titled "Religion as a Caregiving System for Puerto Rican Elders with Functional Disabilities," looks at what role, if any, religion is playing as part of a support system for Puerto Rican elders living in a large New England city. The findings proved troubling for the community and the field of human services.

Food establishments such as grocery stores and restaurants can be found in many Latino communities and are often considered to play a vital role in the life of a community. The chapter titled "Puerto Rican Food Establishments as Social Service Organizations: Results of an Asset Assessment" examines the social service functions of these indigenous institutions and identifies a series of factors for their success. Botanical shops are quite common in Latino communities but are often misunderstood and overlooked by health-related agencies. Chapter 6, "Puerto Rican Elders and Botanical Shops: A Community Resource or Liability?", reports on the results of a key informant survey on the topic.

The last two chapters ("Hispanic Natural Support Systems and the AODA Field: A Developmental Framework for Collaboration" and "Hispanic Natural Support Systems and Alcohol and Other Drug Services: Challenges and Rewards for Practice") are based upon substance abuse prevention research commissioned by the federal government. These chapters provide the reader with an understanding of how natural support systems are manifested within Latino communities and present a developmental framework for engaging these valuable resources.

CONCLUSION

There is little doubt that most practitioners in major urban areas have either experienced or will experience an upsurge in the number of Latinos seeking services. Unless they were fortunate enough to have had the proper training in graduate school, which I believe few have had, they will be ill prepared to address the needs, and the complex and ever-dynamic nature of this population. This book represents an initial step toward redressing gaps in education and experience in graduate school for most researchers and providers of social services. The approaches, issues, rewards, and challenges identified in this book are not restricted to any one profession, region of the country, or urban area. The author hopes that the timeliness of this book makes it relevant for practitioners wishing to better address the needs of this community.

SECTION I: RESEARCH

Chapter 1

Community Asset Assessment and Substance Abuse Prevention: A Case Study Involving the Puerto Rican Community

INTRODUCTION

The human service field has had a long and involved relationship with needs assessments. The professional literature on this topic is rich in theory and case applications, particularly on how needs assessments influence program development (Bell et al., 1983; Humm-Delgado and Delgado, 1986; Marin and Marin, 1991; Marti-Costa and Serrano-Garcia, 1987; McPhillip, 1987). However, this

The author wishes to acknowledge Ms. Carmen Cordero and Maria Salgado, field coordinators; and the youth interviewers.

The research this chapter is based upon was funded through a demonstration grant from the Center for Substance Abuse Prevention (5 H86 SP02208), Rockville, MD, to the Education Development Center, Newton, MA.

This chapter was previously published in *Journal of Child and Adolescent Substance Abuse*, Volume 4(4) 1995.

5

literature has been premised on uncovering unmet needs and has rarely, if ever, taken natural support resources into account in determining need and making programmatic recommendations. This is particularly evident with communities of color—in short, these communities supposedly have prodigious unmet needs and little or no natural resources. This biased perspective, as a result, has serious limitations for the development of culture-specific services that seek to involve significant community sectors (Marin, 1993).

The thrust toward a resiliency/asset model of assessment in the field of substance abuse, as compared to a deficit model, attempts to view community needs within a strength perspective:

> Unfortunately, the dominance of the deficiency-oriented social service model has led many people in low-income neighborhoods to think in terms of local needs rather than assets. . . . The process of identifying capacities and assets, both individual and organizational, is the first step on the path toward community regeneration. Once this new "map" has replaced the one containing needs and deficiencies, the regenerating community can begin to assemble its assets and capacities into new combinations, new structures of sources of opportunity, new sources of income and control, and new possibilities for production. (McKnight and Kretzmann, 1991, pp. 2-3)

Fortunately, there is a growing body of professional alcohol and other drug abuse literature on the importance of culture-specific services based on community assets (Clayton, 1992; Delgado and Humm-Delgado, 1993; Gfroerer and De La Rosa, 1993; Kumpfer, 1987; Newcomb, 1992; Rhodes and Jason, 1988). However, this literature has invariably focused on the development and delivery of services with little or no attention to the process of using community asset/resiliency assessment as a foundation for the development of collaborative services—natural/informal and institutional/formal.

This chapter presents a case example involving an asset assessment of a Puerto Rican community in New England; this research was undertaken by youths (ages thirteen to fifteen) in a substance abuse prevention project. This study is probably one of the first of its kind in the United States and should be of interest to communities/organizations planning to undertake an asset assessment, and to academic settings in preparing future providers/researchers. However, it has implications for other fields and communities of color.

REVIEW OF THE CONCEPTS
OF ASSET/RESILIENCY/NATURAL SUPPORTS

This literature review section will provide the reader with an overview of the concept of resiliency and how it has been operationalized to address the needs of various populations and communities. The emergence of this concept is not new to the field of human services, having been conceptualized in a variety of ways over the past ten years. However, regardless of how this concept has been utilized with various groups (e.g., gender, ethnicity/race, age, socioeconomic class), there have been several themes that are common to all forms of assessment and intervention involving resiliency.

The concept of resiliency has most commonly been operationalized as coping (Eckenrode, 1991), natural support systems (Delgado, 1994, 1995a; Nisbet, 1992), strengths (Davis, 1994; Saleebey, 1992), protective factors (Gfroerer and De La Rosa, 1993; Hawkins, Lishner, and Catalano, 1985), social competence (Freeman, 1990), and community asset/capacity (McKnight and Kretzmann, 1991). However, regardless of how individuals, families, and community strengths are identified, culture is central to the concept.

Cultural pride has been linked with high self-esteem. Thus, the concept of culture forms a central role in the development of a resiliency construct. Resiliency provides a dramatically different alternative to current conceptualizations of risk. Some individuals within a family/community are resilient and able to cope successfully, whereas others cannot. Resilience, in turn, cannot be conceptualized as a fixed attribute of an individual but as vulnerability or protective mechanisms that modify the individual's response to the risk situation and operate at critical points during one's life (Newcomb, 1992; Rhodes and Jason, 1988). Risk-taking behaviors are influenced by a wide range of factors in a community. These factors can be classified as (1) family, (2) peers, (3) psychological, (4) biological, and (5) community (Dryfoos, 1990; Krimsky and Golding, 1992; McWhirter et al., 1993).

However, given that only a relatively small percentage of individuals display risk-taking behaviors, the concept of resiliency and its various manifestations must be taken into account as it plays a central role in the development of substance abuse intervention strategies. In order to move beyond simply identifying and categorizing youth, families, and communities at risk, the focus of any intervention must necessarily shift to understanding the notion of resilience. Rutter (1987) sums up the basis for resiliency as follows:

> Protection does not reside in the psychological chemistry of the moment but in the ways in which people deal with life changes and in what they do about their stressful or disadvantageous circumstances. Particular attention needs to be paid to the mechanisms operating at key points in people's lives when a risk trajectory may be redirected onto a more adaptive path. (p. 329)

Resiliency factors, in essence, are the flip side of risk factors. Newcomb (1992), based upon his work in substance abuse, argues that risk and protective (resilient) factors are in fact endpoints of each. For example, high law abidance (a protective factor) directly limits the likelihood of drug involvement, whereas having many friends/ relatives/ or living in a community with drug pushers (risk factors) directly heightens the probability of drug involvement. In keeping with this perspective, both risk and resiliency factors generally fall into intrapersonal, interpersonal, and community; culture, as already noted, shapes the person-in-environment (ecological), and influences all three perspectives.

The literature on the topic of resiliency notes that high self-esteem and the presence of social supports represent key elements in helping individuals surmount life's trials and tribulations (Caplan and Killilea, 1976; Werner, 1991). The social stress model, for example, views problems as the result of negative long-term outcomes of multiple experiences with significant others and social systems (Albee, 1991). Sullivan (1992) sums up this perspective very nicely:

> A strength perspective . . . offers an alternative conception of the environment. This perspective promotes matching the in-

herent strengths of individuals with naturally occurring resources in the social environment. . . . Recognizing, recruiting, and using these strengths can help maximize the potential of . . . our community. In addition, when the environment is viewed as a source of opportunities . . . rather than an ecology of obstacles, the sheer number of resources we perceive expands dramatically. (pp. 148-149)

Consequently, how we perceive and respond to problems is contingent upon how we feel about ourselves and who/what resources can be used in solving or minimizing the impact of problems. Opportunities, in this instance, must be conceptualized as consisting of both formal and informal (natural).

Davis (1994) and her colleagues have taken a strength/resiliency perspective for examining issues confronting women and in development of gender-specific interventions; these interventions, in turn, are grounded in feminist principles with a strong emphasis on development of self-esteem. Recently, the social context of coping (resiliency) has been receiving much attention from researchers (Eckenrode, 1991). Not surprisingly, their findings have highlighted the importance of viewing coping from a multifaceted perspective with culture playing a central role in the conceptualization and operationalization of the concept. Folkman and colleagues (1991) have utilized the concept of coping in the development and implementation of a coping effectiveness training.

Freeman (1990) has also incorporated the element of coping into her concept of social competence for adolescents; she defines social competence as a lifelong striving toward coping effectively with new developmental challenges. In examining adolescent substance abuse she notes the following:

Any problem, such as adolescent substance abuse for example, can be viewed as an individual's ineffective efforts to achieve a satisfactory level of social competence. This perspective directs attention to multiple factors that can prevent or impair competence in adolescents as well as affect intervention once the lack of competence and substance abuse have become a problem. (p. 247)

The concept of resiliency has also been applied to addressing problems other than substance abuse. Nadel and Morales-Nadel (1993), have taken a resiliency approach to school drop-out prevention among Puerto Rican/Latino youth:

> In order to empower our Puerto Rican/Latino students, we must demonstrate to them the successes and achievements of our community as it has historically struggled to overcome the barriers of prejudice, racism, and linguistic bias. . . . It is going to take a strong, well-developed partnership including home, school, and community to attack the cynicism developed by some of our most promising young people . . . (pp. 154-155)

The authors place a tremendous amount of importance on self-pride and collaboration between all major parties, including those most impacted by the problem.

Rutter (1987) has outlined a four-part framework for examining resiliency among youth, families, and communities:

1. Reduction of negative outcomes by altering the risk or the child's exposure to the risk—for example, restricting alcohol advertisements or liquor establishments in the community.
2. The reduction of a negative chain reaction following risk exposure—providing prenatal care, home support, etc., for adolescents who are abusing drugs.
3. The establishment and maintenance of self-esteem and self-efficacy—cultural pride, refusal skill development.
4. Opening up opportunities for attaining skills/knowledge for success in life—extracurricular involvement, high-quality curriculum development, employment opportunities, i.e., research interviewers.

This framework represents an excellent perspective for developing intervention strategies specifically focused on communities. Holmes (1992), commenting on the importance of involving those being researched and focusing on their strengths, illustrates how the concept of studied resiliency can be operationalized in community-based research:

> Research design should reflect the recognition that those under study have the authority over their lives and possess abilities to

express authority in some way—that they have strengths. Research should focus on eliciting, understanding, and developing these strengths; on how these individuals and groups have surmounted and coped. (p. 159)

The work undertaken by McKnight and Kretzmann (1991) on mapping community capacity (resilient versus deficit/needs), fits well within Rutter's framework. A community that mobilizes the collective resources of its residents increases its chances of winning, and communities are advantaged at the outset when individual residents have more personal resources. Therefore, community mobilization may be one way communities can offset common perceptions of deficiencies in individual resources (Hutcheson and Prather, 1988).

Freeman (1990) proposes increasing the social competence of youth, in this case African American, through training/socialization to seek services from formal sources and natural support systems to prevent or treat substance abuse. Natural support systems have been utilized to reach out to communities of color in a Northern California (Richmond) demonstration project (Delgado, 1995b). This project utilized African-American, Latino (primarily Mexican American, and Southeast Asian (primarily Laotian) natural supports to help substance abusing youth and their families. The Holyoke, Massachusetts, asset assessment study utilized Puerto Rican natural support systems (Delgado and Humm-Delgado, 1982), as the basis from which to identify community informal resources.

The following definition (Delgado, 1994) best sums up the dynamic and important role natural support systems play in Puerto Rican and possibly other Latino communities:

... Natural support systems are composed of a constellation of individuals who relate to you, although not necessarily to each other, on a familiar or even intimate basis. These individuals are an important basis for self-definition and identity formation, and can be assessed freely on a casual basis or for the purposes of meeting specific expressive and/or instrumental needs. The concept of natural support systems extends far beyond the existence of mechanisms that can be utilized as support systems and includes the individuals who *comprise* the support system (i.e., while a church has the potential to be utilized as a natural support system, its utility lies in the personality of its religious leader); consequently, support systems are only as good as the individuals (natural support providers) providing the assistance. Hispanic natural support systems involve extended family members (both related and nonrelated), neighbors, friends, healers, institutions (including religious and other indigenous types), local self-help groups, and community leaders. (pp. 12-13)

The previous definition captures the richness and complexity of Puerto Rican/Latino natural support systems; natural support systems and community are inextricably interrelated.

The use of natural (social) supports, it has been argued, is a form of resiliency by providing an individual/family/community with an opportunity to seek help from informal (culture-based) sources and as a means of reality, testing the nature and severity of circumstances/problems (Eckenrode, 1991). Natural support systems represent indigenous resources that can be used to address expressive and instrumental needs of individuals, families, and communities. These resources are community-based and present opportunities for members of a community to take on help-giving roles (Streeter and Franklin, 1992). Consequently, self-esteem will be enhanced when communities can help themselves. The manifestation of natural support systems will differ based upon community characteristics/ cultural groups.

A group's natural support system is greatly influenced by its beliefs, history, traditions about helping its members as opposed to assistance from outsiders, as well as by the lack of available resources in the larger society (Weber, 1982). The involvement of natural support systems within a comprehensive rubric of resources and services is essential for achieving success in the field of alcohol and other drug abuse (Allen and Allen, 1987). Collaboration between programs, agencies, settings, etc., is not restricted to formal systems but should also involve natural systems. Thus, concepts such as participation, networking, culture, cultural competence, capacity development, community, etc., can be firmly rooted in natural support systems. The Holyoke study, as a result, explored the potential use of natural support systems collaborating with community-based organizations to prevent substance abuse.

DESCRIPTION OF SETTING
AND CONTEXT FOR STUDY

This section will provide the reader with sufficient detail to understand the nature of the setting, rationale for using youth as interviewers, research goals and characteristics of sample population, how the interviewers were prepared for their research tasks, and funding for project.

Description of Site/Interviewers

The community asset assessment described in this study was undertaken during December 1993, in Holyoke, Massachusetts, an industrial city located approximately 100 miles west of Boston. In 1990 it had a population of approximately 44,000, of which 12,700 (28.9 percent) were Puerto Rican; this Latino group constituted 93.5 percent of all Latinos in the city. The Puerto Rican community is young, with a median age of 18, up from 16.4 years in 1980 (The Maurico Gaston Institute of Latino Community Development and Public Policy, 1992). A total of ten Puerto Rican youth (six girls and four boys), aged thirteen to fifteen, conducted the interviews. They, in turn, were supervised by two program facilitators (both Puerto Rican and female) and the director of the project (male Puerto Rican). The youth worked three days per week, approximately three hours per day, for a total of three weeks.

Rationale for Using Youth

Community-based research undertakings in the late 1970s and early 1980s generally agreed that it was important, when feasible, to use Latino youth as interviewers (Bloom and Padilla, 1979; Delgado, 1979, 1981; Padilla et al., 1979; Perez et al., 1980). Although the concept of empowerment was not utilized in presenting key findings from these studies, its presence was central to the research endeavor. Gutierrez (1992) recommends that for this concept to have meaning, it "requires involving members of the ethnic minority community as decision makers with equal power in developing and administering any programs and services" (p. 334).

Consequently, in the spirit of empowerment, Puerto Rican youth were utilized for the following reasons: (1) provide a greater sense of control over the youth's lives, families, and community; (2) instill important research skills and knowledge that will serve youth and the community in future undertakings; (3) provide the community in general, and Puerto Rican community in particular, with a perspective that youth can be, and are vital and contributing members of a community, thus counteracting pervasive views that are deficit-based; and (4) serve as role models for other human service organizations to better utilize youth in service to their community.

Research Goals and Characteristics of Sample Population

The Holyoke study specifically focused on a forty-block area with a very high concentration of Puerto Ricans—this constitutes a major portion of the downtown commercial district and a significant sector of the residential community. This study sought to accomplish four goals: (1) provide a detailed description and location of Puerto Rican natural support systems with a specific focus on houses of worship and merchant/social clubs (grocery stores, botanical shops, etc.); the study did not attempt to identify folk healers and significant community leaders (the former would be very difficult to access without a solid effort of relationship building; the latter because key community leaders had already been identified); (2) provide youth with a resiliency perspective on this community; (3) raise the consciousness of human service organizations/providers concerning positive aspects of the Puerto Rican community; and (4) serve as a basis for a resource directory specifically focused on community assets.

Data were collected on five dimensions: (1) geographical location and category of resource (i.e., commercial, religious, recreational, etc.); (2) listing of key contact person and years in operation; (3) hours/days of operation; (4) type of informal/support services provided (i.e., referral, financial, information, etc.); and (5) general reactions of the interviewer to the receptivity of the institution for collaboration on community activities, projects, etc.

Preparation of Interviewers

The preparation of the field interviewers was based upon work undertaken by Delgado (1979, 1981) in training Latino youth for community-based research. The training addressed six themes: (1) what a community research project involves and why it is important to identify community strengths/resources; (2) description and review of survey instrument (Spanish and English versions), including rationale for question selection and sequencing; (3) discussion role/play of situations when the respondent does not understand the nature of the study/questions or is resistant to answering questions; (4) an exploration of interviewers' feelings/hesitation related to being part of this research project; (5) review of how data will be analyzed and utilized; and (6) discussion of how this study is related to the overall purpose of the Center for Substance Abuse Prevention (CSAP) grant.

The training consisted of a total of six hours of instruction and utilized a variety of teaching methods: (1) didactic; (2) discussion; (3) role play; and (4) group member problem solving. In addition, youth would spend fifteen to thirty minutes at the end of a workday discussing feelings, experiences, and making suggestions to facilitate implementation of the study. These "de-briefing" sessions were informal, unstructured, and were led by the youth themselves.

Funding and Goals for CSAP Project

New Bridges (Nuevo Puente) was a primary prevention project for young Latino (Puerto Rican) adolescents that linked cultural pride and substance abuse prevention. The goals of this CSAP project were: (1) to increase resiliency and protective factors to reduce the likelihood that "high-risk" youth will experiment with and become habitual users of drugs, including alcohol and tobacco; and (2) development of a community-based intervention that enriched and enforced existing substance abuse prevention efforts by promoting acceptance of antisubstance use values and behaviors.

New Bridges utilized a multifaceted approach to substance abuse prevention and targeted various community groups in addition to youth participants. The project developed community and professional advisory committees to aid with the planning and implementation of various trainings and community-sponsored events. Training and consultation were the primary methods used for reaching youth, family, and community leaders. Project youth participants participated in an extensive educational program that stressed cultural awareness (knowledge of Puerto Rican history and culture); academic; study skills; leadership development (conducting workshops and public speaking); alcohol, tobacco, and other drug awareness; and the planning and implementation of community asset assessments. This project received funding for a total of three and a half years and involved active collaboration with a wide range of community-based organizations. Field interviewers were paid $100 for their participation in this research.

PRESENTATION OF KEY FINDINGS

This community-based study consisted of two different phases: (1) identification and (2) interviewing. The identification phase entailed field interviewers, in pairs, identifying all Latino-owned/ operated establishments and filling out a detailed sheet on each setting. This sheet gathered data on the following: (1) name of establishment; (2) address; (3) telephone number if readily available; (4) type of establishment; (5) name of field interviewer; and (6) comments concerning appearance of building/establishment, location, and other pertinent information.

As noted in Table 1.1, a total of thirty-seven establishments were identified for the interview phase. The two most frequently listed establishments were houses of worship (N = 8) and grocery stores (N = 8), followed by clothing stores (N = 6), eating establishments (N = 6), cosmetology settings (N = 2), furniture stores (N = 2), and other (N = 5). The survey, however, did not uncover any social/ hometown clubs or recreational institutions.

It should be noted that the range of institutions went far beyond what is usually expected in a Puerto Rican community, namely, religious, grocery stores, and eating establishments. The Holyoke study noted a radio station, appliance repair shop, clothing stores, beauty parlors, furniture stores, etc. In essence, this extensive range of type of institutions reflect a "maturity" on the part of the community and an increased capacity for providing for a wide range of needs within close geographical proximity.

Twenty-five out of thirty-seven institutions participated in the interview phase of the study. It was not possible to conduct interviews of religious institutions (N = 8) due to evening and weekend

TABLE 1.1. Categories of Establishments Identified and Interviewed

CATEGORY	NUMBER Identified	Interviewed	AVERAGE # OF HRS OPEN	# OF DAYS OPEN
Houses of Worship	8	0	Not Available	Not Available
Bodegas (Grocery Stores)	8	7	13	7
Clothing Stores	6	5	8	6
Eating Establishments	6	4	11	6
Cosmetology Shops	2	2	8	6
Furniture Stores	2	2	9	6
Other: Repair Shop	1	1	8	6
Radio Station	1	1	24	7
Record Store	1	1	10	6
Gift/Party Store	1	1	9	6
Botanical Shop	1	1	9	7
	N = 37	N = 25	X = 10.8	X = 6.4

hours of operation (Delgado and Rosati, 1995); four establishments refused to allow interviews to take place (two eating establishments, one grocery, and one clothing store).

Grocery stores were the most accessible (see Table 1.1), as expected, and were the only institutions, with the exception of a botanical shop and radio station, that were open seven days per week and had the longest hours of operation (thirteen hours per day). The other institutions generally operated Monday through Saturday for approximately nine hours per day.

In examining the length of time in operation (Table 1.2), ten establishments had been in existence one year or less (five less than five months). There were three establishments with a very long history of operation (ten, fifteen, and twenty years); three was the mean number of years all institutions interviewed were in operation. Data are very significant, particularly in light of the large

TABLE 1.2. Years in Operation

PERIOD COVERED	NUMBER OF ESTABLISHMENTS
1 Year or Less	10
1.1 Years to 2 Years 11 Months	6
3 Years to 4 Years	5
5 Years to 10 Years	2
15 Years to 20 Years	2
Mean Number of Years in Operation: 3 Years	

number of business establishments developed during a severe and prolonged economic depression in Massachusetts. This, once again, reflects an increased community capacity to develop infrastructures to meet its own needs. Community capacity development reflects well on a community's ability to build upon and utilize individual, family, and organizational strengths.

Questions pertaining to what kind of assistance these establishments have provided or their willingness to provide information (instrumental or expressive), revealed a wealth of resources targeting people in need. Eighteen institutions stated that people were welcome to come in to converse and not have to purchase goods or services in order to do so. Six institutions provided information on social services and made referrals to social service agencies. Several establishments indicated that they provided crisis counseling (N = 4), food for the hungry (N = 4), loans (N = 3), and credit (N = 6) as needed. One institution (botanical) indicated a willingness to take care of children in case of a crisis. The survey, as a result, revealed an extensive array of social services being provided by these natural support systems.

Twenty establishments noted a willingness to become involved in community events such as festivals, parades, contests, health fairs, and collaborating with human service agencies. Collaboration would take the form of making referrals for services, distributing information, and/or donating food/services/money. In short, these institutions were willing to become more involved with social agencies.

Interviewer comments reinforced the potential for collaboration. Eighteen establishments openly welcomed and validated field interviewer efforts at presenting the community in a positive light, particularly in countering widespread views of rampant drug abuse among Puerto Rican youth. Interviewers also noted the pride expressed by those interviewed of the hard work and dedication it took to establish their businesses and how they wanted to help the community. One institution (radio station) took time to show the youth throughout the establishment. The interviewer's impressions reinforced the receptivity of the institutions to be a part of this research endeavor.

RECOMMENDATIONS

There were many valuable lessons learned from the Holyoke experiences that can help other institutions/communities interested in undertaking an asset assessment. These lessons can best be categorized into the following groupings.

Nature of the Study

Historically, most assessments have generally been needs driven in nature and focused on human service organizations. Consequently, a thrust toward assets and natural support systems is not easily accomplished. Field interviewers often had to spend significant amounts of time describing what was an asset assessment to individuals with minimal or no awareness of the concept of assessment. In addition, many establishments were not aware of the organization undertaking the study. Thus, there was an initial reluctance to participate in this endeavor.

It is recommended that a letter be sent to establishments prior to the interview phase—this was not done in the Holyoke study. This letter, written in English and Spanish, should explain the nature and goals of the study, process, and provide a telephone number they can call to get questions answered. It is also recommended that all Spanish media be contacted to share the nature of the study with the community, in order to minimize fears and confusion concerning the research. It is also strongly encouraged that field researchers start their interviews with establishments that they either know personally or feel comfortable interviewing. The interview of the botanical shop is an excellent case in point. Two interviewers expressed an interest due to familiarity with this institution. Some interviewers did not want to go there for fear of hexes, etc.

Restriction on Days and Times for Interviews

Unfortunately, the use of youth as interviewers does not allow a wide range of hours/days for interviews. Youth are generally restricted to Monday through Friday and after school. Consequently, interviews of religious establishments, for example, could not take place. These institutions were generally open in the evening and on weekends. Several establishments either refused to participate in the study, or required multiple visits, because afternoon periods were the busiest time of the day and taking time away from customers to answer questions was not acceptable. The interviews averaged between fifteen and thirty minutes and this severely limited the number and depth of questions that could be asked. The study, for example, did not gather information on the process or thinking behind the establishment of a business, or what kind of help was made available to facilitate the development of the business.

Resistance to Participation in the Study

This article has already noted a variety of reasons why establishments were either hesitant or refused to participate in this study. The use of youth must be added to the list of reasons. The use of youth can convey a negative message to adults—namely, this is not an important activity, otherwise adults would be doing the interviews. Further, the idea of youth being in a position of "authority" of asking questions may have been a barrier too great to overcome in certain instances. It is important to note, however, that only a small percentage (16 percent) of the establishments refused to participate in the study.

Weather and Season

It is strongly recommended that assessments not be undertaken during the winter months or major holidays (in the Holyoke case,

Christmas). Winter weather is *not* conducive to door-to-door surveys, as it severely hampers scheduling. Several major snowstorms forced major changes in scheduling—canceling certain dates or limiting the amount of interview time; establishments, in many instances, were forced to close. Cold weather, in turn, also limited the amount of time interviewers could be held in the field. Also, several establishments did not want to be bothered during busy holiday periods, the most profitable time of the year. Consequently, fall and spring are perhaps the best seasons for asset assessment.

Supervision/Field Support

As noted, using Latino youth as field interviewers has important implications in planning and implementing a study. However, the use of youth requires more than the usual field support and supervision. The Holyoke study paired youth into twos or threes as a means of increasing mutual support (particularly in those instances where the interviewees did not want to participate), and eliciting and recording information. This makes the process of interviewing expensive, which would not be the case with adult interviewers.

As this study was undertaken in the winter, the weather influenced when interviews could take place; consequently, much time was wasted in transporting youth to various city blocks and waiting to transport them back to the program site. It is recommended that strategic sites be located and used as field bases for interviewers to meet and return to after completing the interviews. It was particularly important that youth have an opportunity at the end of the day to process the events that had transpired. These debriefing sessions, although time-consuming, are particularly important for helping youth put positive and negative experiences into context and to help them problem solve about how to handle particularly distressing situations. For example, there was one instance in which an interviewer entered an especially "dangerous" area of Holyoke and became engaged in a fight. The session at the end of the day was devoted to feelings, alternative strategies to fighting, etc.

Last, it is important for youth to carry identification with them that notes the organization they are working with on the study. Appropriate forms of identification include cards, T-shirts with program emblem, or letters. If the study is undertaken in the summer, T-shirts are particularly effective for conveying this information.

Advisory Committee

Unfortunately, the Holyoke study did not follow the recommendations made by other Latino researchers (Becerra and Zambrana, 1985; Humm-Delgado and Delgado, 1983; Marin and Marin, 1991), namely, establish and fully utilize the advice and services of an advisory committee. Due to very quick planning and startup (end of funding period), there was insufficient time to contact, enlist, and orient members of the Latino community to be part of an asset advisory committee. However, it is strongly recommended that an advisory committee play an influential role in the planning and implementation of an asset assessment. This committee can help in developing appropriate questions for the survey, gaining community access, disseminating publicity about the study, helping in the analysis of results, and most important, taking the results of the study and actively seeking to develop appropriate services. In essence, use of an advisory committee is an important form of empowerment for a community, in addition to making the asset assessment more culture-specific and accepted by the Latino community and community-at-large.

CONCLUSION

The Holyoke study, although not without limitations, represented a significant effort into a new and exciting area of research in the field of alcohol and other drug abuse prevention. In the United States, communities have become more fragmented, resulting in breaks in the naturally occurring linkages among social systems; these linkages provide support and nurturance to individuals and create opportunities for them to participate meaningfully in the community (Bernard, 1990). Further, these linkages help communities define themselves and serve to both reduce unnecessary stress and enhance social competence.

A sense of belonging is found when people feel as if they have been involved in the community change process. This sense of belonging includes an awareness that others will "care," and that the individual has a responsibility and ability to care for the other members of the community. Furthermore, a sense of community engenders meaning and connectedness. Inclusion in the community enables members to create a shared history and common destiny (Allen and Allen, 1987).

The use of natural support systems to help develop and implement substance abuse prevention strategies offers much promise. The Holyoke study highlighted the importance and possibility for bringing greater cooperation and coordination between substance abuse-related organizations and natural support systems. This, however, is not to say that collaboration will take place without great effort and setbacks. Nevertheless, it is not a question of whether, but when collaboration will transpire!

Chapter 2

Puerto Rican Elders
and Gerontological Research:
Avenues for Empowerment
and Participation

INTRODUCTION

The field of gerontology has slowly begun to examine the influence of ethnicity, race, and culture on help-seeking and service utilization patterns (Ball and Whittington, 1995; Barresi and Skinner, 1994; Barresi and Stull, 1993; Coke and Twaite, 1995; Holmes and Holmes, 1995; Stanford and Torres-Gil, 1992). Increased attention to these factors has highlighted the necessity for gerontological organizations to develop services that take into account an elder's cultural context (Capitman, Hernandez-Gallegos, and Yee, 1992).

There is no disputing the need for gerontological organizations to develop a more in-depth and comprehensive understanding of Latino elder social service needs (Bartlett and Font, 1995; Bastida and Lueders, 1994; Espino, 1993; Jimenez and de Figueiredo, 1994). The projected numerical increase in this population is expected to continue well into the twenty-first century (Hayes-Bautista, 1992; Roberts, 1994; Treas, 1995). This increase, in combination with

The author wishes to acknowledge the contributions of all the elders who graciously gave of their time and to Dr. Tennstedt for her review and comments on an earlier draft of this chapter.

This project was funded through a National Institute on Aging Grant (AG11171).

This chapter was previously published in *Activities, Adaptation and Aging*, Volume 21(2) 1996.

25

extensive social needs, will present serious challenges to agencies as they attempt to structure services to meet the needs of this group. Thus, it is imperative that policymakers, planners, and practitioners develop appropriate methods for obtaining data and assessing needs that can be used to develop culture-specific services.

In order to take into consideration the role of culture and how it influences elder perceptions and uses of services (Henderson, 1994; Ragin and Hein, 1993), studies must have a cultural context to guide development of research questions, methodology, and analysis of findings (Delgado, under review, a; Garcia, 1985). In addition, these efforts must also have a set of guiding principles that stress elder assets/resiliency, empowerment, participation, collaboration, and capacity development as a means of involving and benefiting the ultimate beneficiaries of the research—namely, Latino elders and their communities. The field of human services, including gerontology, has not paid sufficient attention to involving communities in the development of services. The above principles serve as guides in translating vision into reality for Latino elders and their communities.

This chapter reports on a series of qualitative-based research activities that were utilized to involve Puerto Rican elders in a large-scale cross-sectional study comparing the disability status and long-term care use of Puerto Rican, African-American and non-Latino white older adults. These activities were implemented to both facilitate and ensure participation of Puerto Rican elders in the study. These activities did serve to maximize participation in all phases of the research and provided avenues for respondent input. This chapter, in addition, will make a series of recommendations to help gerontological organizations undertake assessments (assets and needs), program evaluation, and other forms of service-focused research.

REVIEW OF THE LITERATURE

Recent research literature on Puerto Rican and other Latino elders has examined critical needs and issues related to service delivery (Delgado, 1995; Delgado, under review, b.; Delgado and Tennstedt, under review; Sánchez, 1987; Sánchez-Ayéndez, 1988; Sotomayor and Curiel, 1988). The literature has highlighted several major themes related to active and meaningful participation in all stages of a research process from the conceptualization of research questions to analysis of results (Becerra and Zambrana, 1985; Delgado, in press, a; Marin and Marin, 1991). As discussed elsewhere: "The undertaking of research in urban areas with populations of color, regardless of age, presents a unique set of issues and challenges for researchers . . . there is no aspect of the research endeavor that will not be impacted. . . . The literature, however, is in general agreement that communities being studied must play a role in the research with the nature and intensity of the role depending upon the researcher's level of comfort and philosophical approach towards empowerment" (Delgado, in press, a).

Such involvement of Latino elders, however, has generally been conceptualized as an adjunct activity to quantitative-based survey methods. When used, qualitative-based methods have generally consisted of key informant or focus groups (Marin and Marin, 1991) and have not been part of a multifaceted and systematic approach, or sought to empower elders (Lee, 1994; Marti-Costa and Serrano-Garcia, 1995): "Our greatest challenge lies not in how to effectively research empowerment but how to participate in it and encourage it. A redistribution of actual power is inevitable in order to effectively generate a sense of empowerment" (Chavis and Wandersman, 1990, p. 77). Gerontological organizations, as a result, must be prepared to engage in Latino-oriented research in a manner other than "business-as-usual."

Becerra and Zambrana (1985) have concluded that it is not whether or not there needs to be participation of the Latino community in research endeavors. Rather, it is the degree and nature of their participation that need to be determined. When elders and the community are actively brought into the research process, supports need to be in place to ensure that participation is empowering and meaningful.

DESCRIPTION OF SITE AND STUDY

Springfield, the third largest city in Massachusetts, is located approximately 100 miles west of Boston. It has an overall population of approximately 157,000 residents, of which 26,500 are Latinos (Gaston Institute, 1992). The Latino population is primarily Puerto Rican with approximately 24,000 members (89.4 percent), and elders over the age of sixty-five years old account for approximately 750 (Gaston Institute, 1992).

The research project was funded through a National Institute of Aging grant and investigated ethnic differences among African-American, Puerto Rican, and white, non-Puerto Rican elders in current needs for community-based long-term care, patterns of informal care (natural support systems), and the use of formal services. A total of 591 Puerto Rican elders, 368 of whom indicated having a functional disability, and 214 primary caregivers of those disabled elders were interviewed by telephone or in person (Delgado, under review, b; Delgado and Tennstedt, under review).

DESCRIPTION OF METHODS

The study utilized a multipronged approach to involving Puerto Rican elders and obtaining qualitative data. This model of Latino elder participation consisted of four methods: (1) use of an elder advisory committee (Delgado, in press, a), (2) key informants, (3) focus groups, and (4) a community forum (Delgado, under review, a). As summarized in Table 2.1, each of these methods required different levels of planning, resource intensity, elder involvement, and commitment. Each activity is described in the following text.

TABLE 2.1. Puerto Rican Elder Research Activities

Activity	Planning Phase	Implementation Phase	Analysis Phase
Advisory Committee	(2 Meetings)	(2 Meetings)	(1 Meeting)
Key Informants	(4 Interviews)	(3 Interviews)	(3 Interviews)
Focus Groups	(1 Group)	(1 Group)	(1 Group)
Community Forum			(1 Meeting)

1. *Advisory Committee:* Advisory committees can fulfill a variety of functions related to research and program design. The nature and extent of their role are dependent upon the needs of the organization or researcher. The Springfield Puerto Rican elder advisory commit-

tee consisted of eleven members (nine female and two males) and met a total of five times during the life of the project. This committee assisted the researchers with the following activities: (1) planning (a special focus on question construction, identification of key informants, and interpretations of key informant responses); (2) publicity (identification of sources and assistance in dissemination of information on the project); (3) problem solving (identification of potential respondents and key Latino institutions serving elders); (4) data analysis (interpretation of unexpected findings); and (5) dissemination of findings (assistance with identification of appropriate sources for results to be distributed to).

As a result, the advisory committee played an instrumental role in all facets of the research process by being involved in research design and implementation, as well as shaping the interpretation of data and social service-related recommendations.

2. *Key Informants:* The use of key informants is widely recommended in qualitative-based research. Key informants can be defined as " . . . opportunistically connected individuals with the knowledge and ability to report on community needs . . . because they are important members of their communities, surveying key informants may affect community support for program changes" (McKillip, 1987, pp. 81-82). Names of potential key informants were obtained from the advisory committee and community leaders. Elder key informants were selected because of their leadership roles within the community, or because of their knowledge of elder issues and concerns (Soriano, 1995).

A total of ten Puerto Rican elders were contacted to provide information on a variety of topics: (1) perceptions of key elder needs, (2) identification of indigenous institutions serving elders, (3) interpretation of survey findings, (4) recommendations for service delivery, and (5) assistance with location of elders who may have been missed in sample selection.

3. *Focus Groups:* Like key informants, focus groups are a very popular method for obtaining qualitative data on communities (Krueger, 1988). Focus group can be defined as " . . . an informal, small-group discussion designed to obtain in-depth qualitative information. . . . Participants are encouraged to talk with each other

about their experiences, preferences, needs, observations, or perceptions" (Dean, 1994, p. 339).

A total of three focus groups (each consisting of nine members) were utilized in the Springfield study and scheduled at three different points in the research process. The initial focus group served to orient the researchers to issues confronting Puerto Rican elders and identified potential members for the advisory group. The second focus group helped researchers better understand geographic dispersal of Puerto Ricans within and outside the city. The final focus group assisted in the interpretation of unexpected survey findings.

4. *Community Forum:* A community forum consisting of research respondents (or in the case of a service delivery agency—consumers) has tremendous potential for aiding in interpretation of study findings. According to Witkin and Altschuld (1995) a community forum is a:

> ... general structure, it is analogous to the New England town meeting, in which a community is called together to discuss a pressing issue . . . the community forum (also sometimes called a public hearing, or community speak-up) is used to gather stakeholder concerns or perceptions of need areas, opinions about quality or delivery of services, information on causes of present needs, and exploration of community values. (p. 161)

The Springfield community forum was attended by forty-one elders (thirty-five of whom had participated in the survey) and scheduled during the analysis phase of the research project. The forum sought to accomplish three goals: (1) assistance with interpretation of research findings, (2) suggestions on which community-based organizations should obtain copies of the final report, and (3) recommendations on how findings can influence the structuring of service delivery.

GUIDING PRINCIPLES AND RECOMMENDATIONS

Guiding principles serve an important function by translating vision into action. Principles help guide the development of strategies and activities for involving Puerto Rican and other Latino elders in the information-gathering process, be it "research" or program related. The following principles are interrelated and serve to provide a unified approach for elder involvement (Delgado, 1995).

1. *An asset orientation must form the cornerstone of any effort at elder participation.* The concept of asset has slowly found its way into the human service literature and represents a dramatic shift from a deficit orientation:

> Unfortunately, the dominance of the deficiency-oriented social service model has led many people in low-income neighborhoods to think in terms of local needs rather than assets. These needs are often identified, quantified, and mapped . . . The process of identifying capacities and assets . . . is the first step on the path toward community regeneration. (McKnight and Kretzmann, 1990, pp. 2-3)

This concept, however, is almost totally absent from the gerontological literature and represents a "new" perspective in this field.

An asset-oriented approach to research or service delivery will systematically identify indigenous resources and utilize them in a collaborative effort to meet elder needs. In the Latino community, these assets can take a variety of forms with natural support systems (Delgado, 1995) being the most popular means of operationalizing the concept, and having the greatest promise.

These resources may include a local restaurant that is frequented by Latino elders and can be a site for workshops, conferences, local meetings, etc. (Delgado, in press, c). A grocery may be well known for delivering groceries to elders and can be enlisted to distribute information on services. A local dry goods and clothing store may cater to elders and provide them with credit to purchase goods (Delgado, in press, d). The Latino community may also have botanical shops (cultural pharmacies) frequented by elders and can serve to refer elders for services. Owners of all these establishments can be enlisted to be key informants on elder needs or to participate in focus groups. In essence, the Latino community is a rich source of resources that can be mobilized to work with gerontologists and other helping professions.

2. *Research efforts must develop elder and community capacity as an integral part of participation.* There is no disputing that research or services must be relevant to Latino elders and their communities. However, there is generally little thought or consensus on the role that elder-oriented agencies can play beyond service delivery in the most conventional sense. This principle stresses the need for gerontologists to adapt a capacity-development approach as part of any research and service delivery. Capacity development refers to the use of organizational resources to not only meet presenting needs but also help elders and their communities develop the capacities for self-help.

Capacity development can take the shape of enlisting Latino elders to be part of an advisory committee, project, or organization. Committee members will receive training and support for carrying out their roles. Elders can be recruited, trained, and hired to undertake community-focused workshops on various elder-related topics. With the proper training and support, they can also mount successful public education campaigns. In short, participation in research or other activities must be accompanied with training and support. Once prepared, these elders can transfer newly acquired skills to other arenas or help train other elders.

3. *Data-gathering methods must have multiple goals with participation and empowerment central to any activity or service.* Participation in all aspects of research is a key element in empowering Latino elders. According to Chavis and Wandersman (1990): "Solving problems through voluntary participation in local community institutions and organizations is an American tradition . . . , which is increasingly considered by contemporary policy analysts to be vital for effective urban service delivery" (p. 55). Voluntary participation on the part of Latino elders, as a result, is probably the surest means of ensuring that research will lead to community "ownership" of results, and creation of action to bring necessary changes in service delivery. Empowerment, as a result, is a term much in use in human services, and is achievable when organizations plan *with* rather than *for* Latino elders.

4. *Collaboration between agency and community-based institutions/resources (formal and informal) must always be a part of any research effort.* The human service literature is replete with exam-

ples of collaboration. Organizations derive a tremendous amount of benefit by combining forces and resources in addressing needs. However, gerontological organizations must not restrict their efforts to "formal" community-based institutions. There are numerous natural support institutions such as grocery stores (bodegas), religious organizations (i.e., Catholic, Pentecostal, Seventh-Day Adventist, Jehovah's Witnesses), social clubs, botanical shops (cultural variations of pharmacies), etc., that cater to Latino elders (Delgado, 1995). These institutions, in turn, represent geographical (located within the community), psychological (trust), linguistic/cultural (share similar language and cultural values), and operational (hours and days of operation) accessibility (Delgado, in press, b). Consequently, any form of collaboration cannot help but increase the likelihood of services reaching those in greatest need.

Research must be relevant to elder and community needs with an ultimate focus on restructuring and development of "innovative" service-delivery strategies. The principles addressed above will help guide human service organizations in developing a better working relationship with Latino elders and their communities.

These principles reinforce the importance of flexibility, innovation, and the critical role "nontraditional" settings play in the lives of Latino elders. Heath and McLaughlin (1993) validate these perspectives: "Effective programs often provide activities in nontraditional settings, at nontraditional hours, and with nontraditional personnel, and pay little heed to orthodox boundaries of this service sector, bureaucratic compartments, or professional parameters. The program and the terms on which they are offered take their shape from the needs and contexts of those with whom they work rather than from bureaucratic guidelines, accountability precepts, or objectives formulated at geographic and cultural remove from the local contexts . . . " (p. 62). Researchers must be prepared to engage in activities and enter arenas/settings that are totally new to them!

CONCLUSION

Research and service delivery organizations must develop methods for having elder "voices" heard and taken seriously in the design of projects and services. Qualitative methods hold tremendous promise as vehicles for facilitating elder participation; these methods can also serve to develop elders' capacities to shape services for themselves and their communities.

Latino elder voices have generally not been heard by gerontology institutions. Thus, qualitative methods hold even greater significance for a group that is largely "invisible" and in great need for services. Services for Puerto Rican and other Latino elders must be based upon a heightened awareness of culture and how it influences help seeking.

The Springfield experience has shown that Latino elders have the will and capacity to play instrumental roles in shaping all facets of a research project. There is no question that their participation added significantly to the overall experience of the research team, interpretation of findings, and relevance of the research. But more important, participation served to empower them in their quest to control their destiny in this country.

SECTION II:
ASPECTS OF SERVICE DELIVERY

Chapter 3

Religion as a Caregiving System for Puerto Rican Elders with Functional Disabilities

INTRODUCTION

The presence and utilization of natural support systems by Puerto Rican elders has been highlighted in the professional literature (Cruz-Lopez and Pearson, 1985; Delgado, 1982, 1995; Sánchez, 1987; Sánchez-Ayéndez, 1988); this support system exerts a tremendous influence on elder help-seeking patterns (Delgado, 1997). The family, however, is without question the most important natural support for Puerto Rican elders in the United States and Puerto Rico (Bastida, 1988; Delgado and Tennstedt, pending publication; Gelfand, 1994; Sánchez, 1990; Sánchez-Ayéndez, 1988).

The author wishes to acknowledge Dr. Sharon Tennstedt for her review and comment on an earlier draft of this chapter.

This project was funded through a National Institute on Aging Grant (AG 11171).

This chapter was previously published in *Journal of Gerontological Social Work*, Volume 26(3/4) 1996.

Religious beliefs and practices, as represented through organized religious groups, are undoubtedly ranked closely behind families in influence for many elders (Gaiter, 1980; Gallego, 1988; Sánchez-Ayéndez, 1988). Gelfand (1994) notes the importance of family and church in meeting the needs of elders; the strength of these two institutions, in turn, is very often related to an ethnic group's social history. The African-American church is an excellent case in point (Chatters and Taylor, 1989; Coke and Twaite, 1995; Holmes and Holmes, 1995).

However, contrary to popular opinion, Latinos are not exclusively devout Catholics (Cox, 1995; Niebuhr, 1994); there has been a growing influence of Pentecostal, Seventh-Day Adventist, Jehovah's Witnesses, and Mormons among Puerto Ricans and other Latino groups (Delgado and Rosati, pending publication; Gallego, 1988; Tye, 1994a, b, c, d). This chapter will report on the findings of a study of 558 Puerto Rican elders, 214 of which indicated having a functional disability, and 194 of their primary caregivers in a New England community; the study focused on identifying elder natural support systems and how they are meeting social service needs, with special attention being paid to the role of religion.

OVERVIEW OF THE LITERATURE

This literature review specifically focuses on four dimensions and explore implications for how religion influences Puerto Rican elder help-seeking patterns: (1) definition and role of Puerto Rican natural support systems, (2) religion and Puerto Rican elders, (3) exploration of reasons why new religious groups have made significant inroads into the Puerto Rican/Latino community, and (4) the implications of fundamentalist religion for outreach and services to the community.

Definition and Role of Puerto Rican Natural Support Systems

The professional literature has slowly recognized the importance of natural support systems in the lives of Puerto Rican elders in the United States and Puerto Rico. Various social work scholars, most notably Delgado (1982, 1995), Sánchez (1987), and Sánchez-Ayéndez (1988), have specifically focused on the role of natural support systems in helping Puerto Rican elders meet a range of expressive, informational, and instrumental needs.

Delgado (1995) defines Puerto Rican elder natural support systems as follows:

> Puerto Rican elder natural support systems are a network of individuals, with or without institutional affiliation (family/friends, religious groups, folk healers, and community institutions). They provide assistance (instrumental, informational, expressive) on an everyday basis, as well as in times of crisis, and represent a community's capacity to help itself. Natural support systems also serve as a mechanism for helping Puerto Ricans maintain their cultural heritage. These support systems are accessible (logistically, psychologically, conceptually, and geographically) to all sectors of the community; the assistance provided originates from relationships (familial as well as nonfamilial) that extend beyond the provision of services, but also entail feelings of love, affection, respect, trust, loyalty, and mutuality. In short, natural support systems have responsibility for both giving and receiving assistance. (pp. 118-119)

The foregoing definition of natural support systems touches upon the importance of family, religion, and other sources of support, and stresses their interconnectedness. Puerto Rican natural supports serve as a vehicle for both providing and receiving help in addition to meeting a variety of needs. These systems, in turn, are highly dynamic and may vary from community to community.

Religion and Puerto Rican Elders

There is a paucity of empirical-based articles examining the role of religion in the lives of Puerto Rican elders in the United States and Puerto Rico (Gallego, 1988). The Hartford study remains one of the few published research efforts in this area and reported on several important findings: (1) Faith is viewed as a critical element in an elder's life (84 out of 85 answered in the affirmative), (2) Puerto Rican elders were not attending church as often compared with previous years (31.8 percent), and (3) Females consider themselves more religious than males (41 percent consider themselves very religious compared to 23 percent for males).

Several articles, theoretical in nature, have identified why religion must be considered as part of an elder's natural support system (Bartlett and Font, 1994; Delgado, 1982; Sánchez, 1987). Religious support fulfills spiritual as well as more "earthly" needs for elders. Religion as a support system increases in significance for Puerto Rican elders who have left Puerto Rico and settled in the United States, finding themselves increasingly more isolated from family and community.

Exploration of Reasons Why New Religious Groups Have Made Significant Inroads into the Puerto Rican/Latino Community

No study of religious influence on Puerto Ricans/Latinos can ignore the dramatic changes that are occurring in the community. A recent analysis of the increase in popularity of non-Catholic (fundamentalist) religious groups among Latinos noted that various religions have undertaken significant recruitment efforts targeting this population:

> About 2.7 million Mormons, or nearly 31 percent of the church's 8.7 million members, live in Mexico and Central and South America, according to the church's 1993 statistics . . . in 1980 . . . the church had about 700,000, or about 15 percent of its 4.6 million members worldwide . . . from 1970 to 1993, the number of people in Latin America and the Caribbean who were members of Assemblies of God churches grew from about 2.2 million to 16.5 million. . . . (Niebuhr, 1994, p. 36)

Delgado and Rosati (pending publication), in their analysis of the impact of fundamentalist religious groups in the Puerto Rican/Latino community, identify five key factors for their popularity:

1. These religious groups have sought to maintain the Puerto Rican culture as central part of the ministry through the use of the Spanish language, holidays, food, etc.
2. These institutions provide a setting that supports the family and helps them make the necessary adjustments to life in the United States.
3. A conscious effort is made to provide for the spiritual and physical needs of the congregation through provision of social

services, adult education, recreational activities, and possibilities of assuming leadership roles in the church (Caraballo, 1990).

4. Ministers are Puerto Rican/Latino and often represent the same socioeconomic class as the congregation, minimizing social distance.

5. Churches are located in the community, and are accessible geographically and psychologically.

The influence of religious fundamentalists has taken on greater significance for Puerto Rican elders residing in the United States. Stevens-Arroyo and Stevens-Diaz (1993) provide an explanation as to why non-Catholic religious groups offer Puerto Ricans and other Latino groups greater access and acceptance:

> The difficulties placed in the way of the practice of Catholicism by prejudiced clergy or parishioners often rendered it more attractive to the Spanish-speaking in urban centers to join Pentecostal and Evangelical churches. Less burdened by institutional interests, open to a married clergy, and able to adapt quietly to social conditions, these other religions experienced considerable success recruiting Latino members in virtually every urban center of the United States. Usually close-knit groups consisting of a few extended families, such churches offered Latinos an intensity of religious experience that was hard to come by in a segregated Catholicism. (p. 244)

Caraballo (1990), in her dissertation on the topic of Pentecostal ministers in Boston, Massachusetts, makes similar observations to those of Stevens-Arroyo and Stevens-Diaz (1993) concerning the social role fulfilled by churches. These churches are generally led by ministers who reflect the cultural and socioeconomic status of the congregation; they speak the same language, live in and know their community, and represent their congregations' values.

Implications of Fundamentalist Religion for Outreach and Services

The literature identifies a wide range of services that are provided by fundamentalist churches across the United States. Delgado and Rosati (pending publication), noted an average of 7.3 types of social services provided by eleven Pentecostal churches in Holyoke, Massachusetts. Caraballo (1990) noted that these religious leaders also functioned as social workers, information-referral specialists, interpreters, and providers of transportation. In short, the spiritual dimension of their position was closely tied to that of a social service provider.

In summary, the professional literature has raised the importance of religion in the lives of Puerto Rican elders; religion meets spiritual, as well as expressive and instrumental needs; the literature also identified a growing membership in non-Catholic religious affiliations. Last, religious institutions can be expected to play an influential role in meeting Puerto Rican elder spiritual and social needs.

METHODS

Research Questions: The study sought answers to four important questions: (1) Are fundamentalist Puerto Rican elders more likely than their Catholic counterparts to consider themselves quite religious?; (2) To what extent are religious institutions, particularly fundamentalist churches, assuming caregiver roles for Puerto Rican elders?; (3) To what extent are religious institutions, particularly fundamentalist churches, providing organized group activities for Puerto Rican elders?; and (4) Are fundamentalist Puerto Rican elders more likely than Catholics to have access to multiple caregivers?

Sample: The study sample of Puerto Ricans is drawn from the Springfield Elder Project, a comparative observational study to investigate the needs for assistance with daily living activities and the sources (formal and informal), and patterns of this help within and between African American, Puerto Rican, and white, non-Puerto Rican elders over age 60. The study was located in Springfield, Massachusetts, for the following reasons: (1) the older population is socioeconomically diverse; (2) the city has sufficiently large populations of older African Americans and Puerto Ricans; and (3) because the city is a major point of population dispersal for Puerto Ricans, they comprise almost all of the Latino population in the city. This permitted the study to focus on one Latino subgroup in order to avoid obscuring any between-group differences that could result from variability in Latino culture.

Data Collection: Interviews with elder respondents were conducted primarily by telephone in either English or Spanish. English-Spanish equivalents of the survey instruments were developed using back translation techniques (Becerra and Shaw, 1984; Lindholm, Marin, and Lopez, 1980). In-home interviews were conducted when necessary (31 percent of the Puerto Rican cases), typically for persons without a telephone or with a nonpublished telephone number. Proxy interviews were conducted when the elder was too functionally or cognitively impaired to complete the interview. Both in-home and proxy interviews were conducted more frequently with Puerto Rican respondents than with the other two groups.

A two-stage design was used. In the *first stage,* data were collected from the older persons. Respondents were first screened for functional disability. If not disabled, a brief (i.e., fifteen-minute) interview was conducted collecting sociodemographic data and information regarding their natural support system to investigate potential sources of informal care.

Elders identified as functionally disabled (self-reported difficulties in 1 of 13 daily living activity areas) received a more extensive interview, collecting data regarding their informal caregiving network (number of relatives, relationship, age, gender, proximity, frequency of contact), the types of help provided by these caregivers (e.g., personal care, housing, shopping, cooking, house maintenance, transportation, financial management, arranging services) and their use of formal long-term care services. If receiving informal care, the name, address, and telephone number of the person providing the *most* help (i.e., the primary caregiver) was gathered.

In the *second stage,* telephone interviews were conducted with the primary informal caregiver. Detailed data regarding the types and amount of help provided were collected from the caregiver. Sociodemographic data about the primary caregiver and other (i.e., secondary) caregivers, cultural factors, the motivation for providing care, and the impact of this care on their lives were also collected.

Analysis: To describe this population of Puerto Rican elders, caregivers, and the caregiving arrangement, univariate (frequency distributions, means) and bivariate (chi-square) statistics were used.

Variables considered in the analyses included elder characteristics: age, gender, disability, religious affiliation, level of religiosity, organized group participation, residence (with caregiver or not), number of caregivers, and socioeconomic status (SES); and caregiver characteristics: relationship to elder, gender, marital status, and employment status. In addition, the following characteristics of the caregiving situation were considered: number of caregivers, reasons for assuming and continuing in the caregiver role, and the number of potential caregivers.

Finally, the hours of care per week were collected for several types of informal care and community services. Services purchased privately in addition to those provided by public and private agencies were considered formal services to capture more completely the use of formal care. Hours per week for each type of informal care and formal services were summed to obtain total hours per week of informal and formal care, respectively.

FINDINGS

This section presents data on five key aspects: (1) a brief demographic profile of Puerto Rican elders, (2) religion of elders, (3) organized group participation of elders, (4) elder primary caregivers, and (5) religious affiliation and caregiver availability.

Profile of elders: The Puerto Rican elder population in Springfield, Massachusetts, has an average age of 70.7 and has resided in the United States for a considerable period of time; 41.2 percent had resided in the United States between ten and thirty years and 48 percent more than thirty years. The average period of residence in Springfield, however, was close to nineteen years (18.85), with approximately 21 percent stating thirty years or more.

As noted in Table 3.1, Puerto Rican elders receiving informal care were quite disabled, with approximately 50 percent living with their caregiver (Delgado and Tennstedt, under review). Those elders who did not live with their caregivers still had to have almost daily contact with them (76.5 percent); almost 60 percent (61.7 percent) had daily telephone calls, with an additional 12 percent calling several times per week.

Religion of elders: Puerto Rican elders generally considered themselves either quite religious (60.1 percent) or as religious as others (28.5 percent); only 11.5 percent considered themselves as

TABLE 3.1. Characteristics of Care Recipients (n = 214)

	n	%	Mean	S.D.
Gender: Female	134	62.6		
Age (Range 60-105)			70.7	8.1
60-64	41	26.2		
65-74	107	50.0		
75+	66	23.8		
Marital Status: Married	68	31.8		
SES (Range 0-100)			27.5	19.3
Number Disabilities			6.8	3.2
(Range 0-13)				
Health Status:				
Very Good/Good	18	8.4		
Fair	119	55.6		
Poor	77	36.0		
Co-Resides with Caregiver	103	48.1		

having little or no religion. Nevertheless, there were significant differences in how this question was answered for Catholics and fundamentalists.

As noted in Table 3.2, fundamentalists had a greater tendency than Catholics to consider themselves quite religious. This finding was expected based upon a review of the literature. Of the 224 Puerto Rican elders who noted they were religious, i.e., "Quite religious" or "About like others," 57.1 percent (N = 128) stated they were Catholic followed by Pentecostals with 26.3 percent (N = 59), and other fundamentalist groups (Jehovah's Witnesses, Seventh-Day Adventist, and other groups) with 16.5 percent (N = 37).

Organized group participation of elders: A relatively small (16.8 percent) group of elders who indicated having a disability (N = 48) indicated that they belonged to organized groups, clubs, or organizations. A higher number of elders were expected to be a part of formalized groups, particularly since religious affiliation was very high.

As noted in Table 3.3, there were significant differences according to religious affiliation. Catholics represented a majority (N = 33) of those indicating participation in an organized group (66.8 percent),

TABLE 3.2. Comparison by Religious Denomination

	Catholic		Pentecostal		Other		x^2	d.f.	p
	n	%	n	%	n	%			
How Religious:							16.38	4	<.01
Quite religious	75	50.0	48	77.4	29	70.7			
About like others	53	35.3	11	17.7	8	19.5			
Little or not at all	22	14.7	3	4.8	4	9.8			
Attend Groups: Yes	33	19.8	8	10.8	7	15.6	3.00	2	ns
Number of Caregivers:							15.70	6	<.05
0	79	47.3	24	32.4	17	37.8			
1	48	28.7	28	37.8	11	24.4			
2	24	14.4	15	20.3	16	35.6			
≥3	16	9.6	7	9.5	1	2.2			

TABLE 3.3. Characteristics of Caregivers (n = 194)

	n	%	Mean	S.D.
Gender: Female	155	79.9		
Age			51.2	15.6
Relationship to Elder[a]				
Spouse	50	26.5		
Offspring	103	54.5		
Other-Relative	28	14.8		
Non-Relative	8	4.2		
Marital Status: Married	96	49.5		
Employment Status: Unemployed	145	74.7		
Duration of Caregiving: Years			7.1	7.6
Number of Caregivers				
1	99	51.0		
2	41	21.2		
3+	54	27.8		

[a]n = 189

followed by Pentecostals (N = 8) with 16.7 percent and other funda-mentalist groups (N = 7) with 14.6 percent.

Elder primary caregiver: Table 3.3 shows that the average elder had one primary caregiver (51.0 percent). Nevertheless, a number of elders had two (21.2 percent) or three (27.8 percent).

As indicated in Table 3.3, family members accounted for over ninety percent (95.8 percent) of an elder's primary caregivers, with daughters being the most frequently mentioned caregiver. Formal providers and nonrelatives accounted for just 4.2 percent. Formal and religious caregivers were noticeable by their absence. The lack of formal services in the elders' lives was expected. However, the minimal role of religious institutions was not, particularly since a high percentage of elders belong to fundamentalist churches.

Affiliation and caregiver availability: As noted in Table 3.3, there were significant differences between religious affiliation and whether or not an elder indicated he or she had someone to turn to for help if needed. It was expected that fundamentalist religious groups would, when compared to Catholics, have a greater social network of poten-tial caregivers if needed. However, this was not the case, with Catho-lics having a higher percentage of potential caregivers.

Catholic elders consistently had a higher percentage of potential caregivers in each of the three categories with Pentecostals general-ly having more than other fundamentalist groups, with the category of two potential caregivers being the exception.

DISCUSSION OF FINDINGS

Unfortunately, the lack of data on the role of religion in the lives of Puerto Rican and other Latino elders makes comparisons very difficult to make. While a complete census was attempted through the sampling strategy, the analysis is limited to Puerto Ricans who have migrated and stayed in the United States. This group, as the literature has reported, tends to be less formally educated and eco-nomically poorer than elders who never left the Island. Consequent-ly, generalizations can only be made to Puerto Ricans residing in midsized urban areas of the United States. The findings from the Springfield study, nevertheless, raised important issues and consid-erations regarding the role of religion in meeting Puerto Rican elder social service needs.

The Hartford study of Puerto Rican elders indicated that 72.9 percent (N = 62) were Catholic, 22.3 percent (N = 18) Pentecostal, and 5.2 percent (N = 5) other (Gallego, 1988). The religious affiliation breakdown was not too dissimilar from those found in Springfield.

The high percentage of Catholics, however, was not unexpected. Nevertheless, Pentecostals and other religious groups have made significant inroads into the Puerto Rican community in the United States.

The social needs of Puerto Rican and other Latino elders have been well documented (Bastida and Lueders, 1994). In addition, Puerto Rican elders residing in the United States generally do not possess a high level of English language skills, increasing the likelihood of experiencing isolation and marginalization in this society. Religion, as a result, represents an arena where elder needs can be met within a cultural and community context, safeguarding their self-respect.

If the trend of fundamentalist religious group outreach into Puerto Rican/Latino communities continues for the rest of this century and into the twenty-first century (Cox, 1995), there are tremendous implications for how social service organizations can reach and serve elders. These religious institutions, as a result, can be expected to assume greater influence over elders and their primary caregivers.

As already noted in the definition of Puerto Rican elder natural supports, these systems are interconnected, and any intervention involving natural supports must not be undertaken until there has been an in-depth assessment (Cruz-Lopez and Pearson, 1985):

> . . . it is important for human service workers to be aware that any intervention involving these informal support systems as an adjunct to formal helping efforts must be carefully planned and implemented lest a misdirected effort interrupt the effectiveness of informal support networks. (p. 486)

Quite unexpectedly, religious organizations played a minimal role in providing care for Puerto Rican elders who indicated they needed it. The literature had highlighted the importance of religious institutions, particularly Pentecostals and other non-Catholic groups, in helping elders meet a variety of social needs.

Fundamentalist groups have been widely credited with providing a multitude of services that go beyond those usually associated with religious institutions. These services, in turn, have played a critical role in the recruitment of new members. Consequently, the Springfield study expected to find Pentecostals and other fundamentalist groups playing a prominent role in the lives of elders. Instead, the data provide a picture of religious organizations that have almost exclusively focused on the spiritual needs of Puerto Rican elders, and left social service needs to be met by family and formal providers.

An examination of the African-American church and its relation to elders provides an important context for developing a better understanding of why Puerto Rican religious institutions, particularly those that are fundamentalist, have not played a more prominent caregiver role in Springfield.

Holmes and Holmes (1995) comment that in addition to "social spiritual" fulfillment, African-American elderly derive economic aid from the congregation. Coke and Twaite's (1995, p. 63) analysis of the literature on the role of the African-American church in elders' lives notes that they benefit directly and indirectly: "(1) derive satisfaction directly from their religious faith; (2) benefit directly from the social interaction with church membership; and (3) benefit indirectly from the social interactions that are associated with church-related social events."

Blackwell (1985) identifies seven significant functions of the African-American church:

> (1) it provides a cohesive institutional structure within the black community; (2) it is an instrument for the development of black leadership; (3) it is a base for citizenship training and community social action; (4) it performs major educative and social roles; (5) it acts as a charitable institution; (6) it is an agency for the development of black business structures or ventures; and (7) it serves as an index of social class. (p. 26)

Hamilton (1972) adds a different dimension to Blackwell's list by highlighting the role of the preacher as a civic as well as spiritual leader, counselor, friend, and social worker. He also stresses the impossibility of separating the preacher from the church itself:

The black preacher is, for the most part, a passionate figure in the lives of black people. He intends to be; his people want him to be; and it would be straining to achieve almost an unnatural condition to make it otherwise. (p. 3)

A comparison of the African-American church with Puerto Rican fundamentalist churches uncovered some striking similarities: (1) both have ministers who are indigenous to the community, (2) both provide cohesion to the community, (3) both perform major educative and social roles, and (4) both are charitable institutions. However, there are major differences, particularly in how Puerto Rican churches view their mission toward social and economic justice: (1) they generally do not undertake social action campaigns; (2) development of business structures and ventures are not part of their mission; (3) leadership development, if undertaken, is internally directed and focused on institutional roles; and (4) they do not function as an index of social class.

Most of the literature, particularly newspaper articles, examined Puerto Rican fundamentalist groups in large urban areas of the United States. The results of the Springfield study may reflect the influence of urban size, or a developmental stage in how these institutions assume caregiver roles for elders and other age groups. Namely, the "newer" fundamentalist churches concentrate on meeting spiritual needs. However, after an initial phase devoted to this goal, they then move on to social needs of the congregation. This may explain the minimal role religion has played in meeting Puerto Rican elder needs. Unfortunately, data were not gathered on religious institutions in the community to help answer this question.

Religious institutions can develop closer ties with formal organizations as a means of helping family caregivers relieve the burden of care. This relationship can be facilitated by the absence of social service provision within churches, thus minimizing "turf" conflicts. However, although they share much in common with African-American churches, where considerable collaborative efforts with social service organizations have transpired, their congregation and leaders are also very dissimilar (i.e., different culture, language, and "newness" to this country).

IMPLICATIONS FOR SOCIAL WORK PRACTICE

The results of the Springfield study have raised important implications for social work practice with Puerto Rican elders. Gelfand (1994) notes that elder newcomers to the United States can often find a point of entry into a community through a house of worship. Churches, as a result, can be an excellent setting to reach out to support, provide information on social services and entitlements, and orient an elder to a community's natural support system. A church serves as a means of providing continuity between a point of departure (homeland) and a new destination.

However, social service organizations wishing to reach Puerto Rican and other Latino elders cannot automatically assume that churches will welcome their outreach. Fundamentalist churches rarely have a long and positive working relationship with mainstream social service organizations, and may be distrustful of their intentions (Delgado and Rosati, forthcoming publication). The process of developing a working relationship with these institutions can be facilitated if a social service setting enlists the support of a Latino community-based organization to help broker an agreement.

The Springfield results indicate a population in great need of services with a very limited caregiving system, with churches not being major providers of services. Consequently, if these findings are applicable to other similar-sized urban areas, social service agencies are in a propitious position to reach a population that is usually considered "isolated" from mainstream society. Social service organizations, in turn, must be prepared to engage in a relationship-building process before they can actually have churches collaborate with them in service delivery.

Social service agencies must also endeavor to reach out to the caregivers as a means of supporting a system of care that can easily be overwhelmed by the needs of elders (Sánchez, 1987). Caregivers, too, have tremendous needs that must be addressed in order to better serve elders. In short, social workers must endeavor to work in partnership with primary caregivers, churches, and other natural support systems. A strength/resiliency/asset perspective in this community will dictate a service delivery strategy predicated on supporting, building upon, and enhancing indigenous resources whenever possible (Saleebey, 1992).

Churches are invariably located within the community, providing easy access to elders and their primary helpers. In addition, these settings are nonstigmatizing and facilitate provision of counseling, development of support groups, information and referral, literacy campaigns, and other services in an atmosphere that values Puerto Rican culture. However, before churches provide space, accessibility, and support, they must trust and respect the agency and its personnel.

Churches have not only survived but expanded in membership and must be considered seriously in any effort at outreaching and serving Puerto Rican and other Latino elders. The potential for collaborative projects is great if social service agencies are willing to give these institutions the respect they would accord any other formal institution that has embraced community participation and achieved a high degree of consumer legitimacy.

CONCLUSION

The Springfield study raised important implications pertaining to the role of religious institutions in meeting Puerto Rican elder health and social service needs. Although fundamentalist religious groups have a significant presence in the community, they are not significant providers of social services for elders. The lack of services, however, may be a phenomenon restricted to Springfield, Massachusetts. However, if this is not the case, it has tremendous implications for how Puerto Rican elders can meet their health and social service needs in the United States.

Social service organizations can no longer view service delivery to Puerto Rican and other Latino elders from a narrow perspective with elders in need coming to the agency. It is necessary to broaden the arena of service provision to include the community and its natural support systems. Religion may or may not be a key provider of social services. However, regardless of the answer to this question, these institutions must be seriously considered in any service delivery to elders.

Chapter 4

Puerto Rican Food Establishments as Social Service Organizations: Results of an Asset Assessment

A tremendous need exists for the social work profession to re-examine service delivery to communities of color in the United States. Recent interest in identifying and utilizing community assets represents an important shift in paradigms concerning undervalued communities in general, and communities of color in particular (Kretzmann and McKnight, 1993; McKnight and Kretzmann, 1991; Rutter, 1987). Traditional social service approaches that emphasized needs and deficits have not resulted in empowering communities (Cross, 1988; Delgado, pending review; Gutierrez and Ortega, 1991; Gutierrez, Ortega, and Suarez, 1990; Mason, 1994).

These approaches have generally been premised upon the assumption that communities do not have the capacity, desire, or resources to help themselves. Consequently, it is necessary for outside sources to provide guidance, moral support, and resources to meet local needs. These approaches are not only disempowering, but also narrow in how they conceptualize resources, i.e., formal (Allen and Allen, 1987; Daley and Wong, 1994; Delgado and

The author wishes to acknowledge the two anonymous reviewers whose insight and suggestions made this chapter more relevant for community practice.

The research this chapter is based upon was funded through a demonstration grant from the Center for Substance Abuse Prevention (5 H86 SP02208), Rockville, MD, to the Education Development Center, Newton, MA. The author was principal investigator on this grant.

This chapter was previously published in *Journal of Community Practice*, Volume 3(2) 1996.

Rosati, pending review; Florin and Wandersman, 1990; Glugoski, Reisch, and Rivera, 1994).

The Latino community in the United States serves as an excellent example of how indigenous resources (natural support systems) can be utilized in the planning and delivery of human services (De La Rosa, 1988; Delgado, 1994; Delgado, pending publication, a; Delgado and Humm-Delgado, 1982; Suarez, 1992). The Latino community, although not homogenous in composition (Castex, 1994; U.S. Bureau of the Census, 1991), has a rich cultural tradition of helping. Consequently, the challenge for human services is how to identify and engage these cultural resources.

This chapter examines one source of resources, food establishments (grocery stores and restaurants), and the multiple roles they play in helping one Latino group (Puerto Rican). An asset assessment of a Puerto Rican community in a New England city is described and the results analyzed from the perspective of developing collaborative activities/projects between these forms of natural support systems and human service organizations.

It is necessary, however, to pause and examine the implications of utilizing "self-help" and "natural support systems" concepts with undervalued communities such as the one addressed in this article. Concepts such as the aforementioned are receiving a great deal of attention at the national and local levels. Both the political "right" and "left" have stressed the importance of empowering communities as an approach for meeting social economic needs. Nevertheless, the manner in which empowerment practices are operationalized and the meaning they have for government intervention, will vary depending on one's political perspective.

This chapter takes the stance that government intervention/resources are essential in helping marginal communities mobilize to meet their own needs. However, these resources must not undermine "natural" helping systems, and instead, must be provided as adjuncts to or in collaboration with indigenous resources. Government intervention/resources, as a result, cannot succeed in helping undervalued communities without taking into account a "community's capacity" to help itself; however, a community cannot be expected to rely totally upon itself without outside resources. In sum, a partnership is necessary for communities to be successful in meeting current and future needs.

THEORETICAL FOUNDATION

A variety of theoretical approaches in the community organization literature lend themselves to analysis of Puerto Rican food establishments and their role in the community; however, the concepts of "free space" and "urban sanctuary" are theoretical approaches that are complementary in a variety of ways and applicable to the topic of this chapter.

The concept of "free spaces" developed by Evans and Boyte (1986) serves as an excellent conceptualization for examining Puerto Rican food establishments and other natural support systems. They state:

> The central argument . . . is that particular sorts of public places in the community, what we call free spaces, are the environments in which people are able to learn a new self-respect, a deeper and more assertive group identity, public skills, and values of cooperation and civic virtue. Put simply, free spaces are settings between private lives and large-scale institutions where ordinary citizens can act with dignity, independence, and vision. (p. 17)

According to the authors, families, and places such as beauty parlors, barber shops, social/civic organizations, houses of worship, and other indigenous organizations (owned and controlled by those who are oppressed), are settings where individuals can come into contact and interact with others in similar circumstances.

Puerto Rican food establishments, as will be noted, are not large institutions with a high volume of business. Nevertheless, they represent one of the few economic or social institutions that are owned, staffed, and patronized by the community. These settings, like the free spaces analyzed by Evans and Boyte (1986), can help facilitate customer exchange of ideas and experiences with social injustices, etc., and assist them in translating these sentiments and experiences into community organization, resistance, and social action.

Marginalized communities have few settings and opportunities to come together to discuss common concerns and needs; free spaces represent vehicles for expression and action that are not controlled by "elites." In essence, indigenous institutions, whether for- or nonprofit, provide a free space for communities to organize and provide services that go beyond what is typically expected, and in a manner that stresses self-respect.

A critique of the concept of free spaces (Fisher and Kling, 1987, p. 43) highlights the notion that social action may not originate from these settings: "We find the work of Harry Boyte and Sara Evans to be valuable regarding the necessary role of free spaces, but disagree with the idea that such spaces are, of themselves, the prime factors of movement building."

Although the potential exists for social change and reform, Puerto Rican food establishments have, instead, served to provide a variety of social services to a community with great needs and few "formal" resources/organizations, and have not played a critical role in galvanizing the Puerto Rican community of Holyoke into social action.

The concept of urban sanctuary articulated by McLaughlin, Irby, and Langman (1994) is complementary with Evans and Boyte's free spaces and also finds "currency" in application to Puerto Rican food establishments. Although the authors do not make specific reference to Evans and Boyte's research and scholarship, the use of urban sanctuary spaces is set within a community/cultural context with implications for social action.

McLaughlin, Irby, and Langman's work focused on violence and inner-city youth who are oppressed as a result of class and race/ethnicity; they stressed the importance of creating a safe and meaningful context (space) where these youths could meet; exchange ideas, histories, etc.; and result in the creation of an environment that is responsive to their needs. The authors further comment on the concept of space (pp. 212-213): " . . . organizations and activities, while well intentioned, are disappointments to youth . . . they fail because they provide a space for you to be in, not a place for you to be."

The establishment of a network of concerned community members, providers, and organizations (the latter of which include indigenous resources and institutions) is necessary for action to have meaning within a community context. Puerto Rican food establishments are settings where the community is accepted without fear of experiencing discrimination based on socioeconomic class and ethnicity; business transactions and personal interactions transpire within a "safe" environment with cultural meanings and symbols. These sanctuaries—free spaces—must be prepared to meet a wide range of community needs if they are going to thrive and be accepted by the community.

REVIEW OF THE LITERATURE

The importance of reaching out to those in need within the confines of the community has been well documented, particularly with groups whose primary language is not English (Gutierrez and Ortega, 1991; Gutierrez, Ortega, and Suarez, 1990). Community, however, is a construct that is not restricted to civic, religious, or human service agencies; this construct must also cover indigenous, or natural institutions and systems (Collins and Pancoast, 1976; Gottlieb, 1981, 1988; Pearson, 1990; Whittaker and Garbarino, 1983).

The presence and utilization of natural support systems represent an important dimension in the help-seeking patterns of Puerto Ricans and other Latino groups (Delgado and Humm-Delgado, 1982; Sánchez, 1988; Sánchez-Ayéndez, 1987; Valle and Vega, 1980). The definition of Puerto Rican natural support systems developed by Delgado (pending publication, a) will serve as the basis for analysis and description in this article:

> Puerto Rican . . . natural support systems are a network of individuals, with or without institutional affiliation (family/friends, religious groups, folk healers, and community institutions). They provide assistance (instrumental, informational, and expressive) on an everyday basis as well as at times of crisis, and represent a community's capacity to help itself. Natural support systems also serve as a mechanism for helping Puerto Ricans maintain their cultural heritage. These support systems are accessible (logistically, psychologically, conceptually, and geographically) to all sectors of the community; the assistance provided originates from relationships (familial as well as nonfamilial) that extend beyond the provision of services, but also entail feelings of love, affection, respect, trust, loyalty, and mutuality. In short, natural support systems have responsibility for both giving and receiving assistance. (pp. 118-119)

The framework developed by Delgado and Humm-Delgado (1982), which categorized natural support systems as falling into four categories (family/close neighbors/friends; religion; folk healers; merchant/social clubs), lends itself for examining grocery stores (bodegas/cormados) and restaurants; food-related institutions fall under the category of merchant/social clubs. This category consists of institutions, profit and nonprofit, that are community-based, and are staffed, patronized, and owned by community residents. These institutions (free spaces/urban sanctuaries), in turn, fulfill a variety of important roles that go beyond the selling of merchandise or providing recreational services.

Puerto Rican bodegas and restaurants have received only minimal attention in the social work/human service literature (De La Rosa, 1988; Delgado and Humm-Delgado, 1982; Sánchez, 1988; Vazquez, 1974), even though they are a very significant force in Puerto Rican communities across the United States. Historically, bodegas were the nucleus of a neighborhood, serving as a focal point for residents (Korrol, 1983). Howe (1986, p. 8) notes: "The bodega was the first economic base of the community, a way for the family to stay together and feel independent . . . the bodega was like part of the extended family, where everybody knew each other. . . . " Bodegas have been estimated to provide at least 50 percent of the food marketed to Puerto Ricans/Latinos in this country (Agins, 1985; Fitzpatrick, 1987; Howe, 1986).

These institutions fulfill a variety of important functions within the community and meet a unique set of needs. Aldrich and Waldinger (1990, p. 115), in their analysis of why ethnic enterprises succeed, note the unique position indigenous commercial institutions have within their respective communities: " 'The protected market hypothesis' . . . posits that the initial market for ethnic entrepreneurs typically rises within the ethnic community itself. If ethnic communities have special sets of needs and preferences that are best served by those who share those needs and know them intimately, then ethnic entrepreneurs have an advantage." Serving the special needs of the community, as a result, extends beyond providing a product; there is also the provision of services that have cultural meaning. These needs can be conceptualized along instrumental, expressive, and informational spheres. However, they generally fall into three major categories: (1) provision of employment for local residents (Burros, 1990; Levine, 1990; Raynor, 1991; Rierden, 1992; Sarason and Koberg, 1994; Terry, 1992); (2) opportunity for opening small businesses (Carmody, 1972; Gonzalez, 1992; Hernandez, 1994; Rohter, 1985a; Stout, 1988); and (3) provision of a wide range of personal/social services (Vazquez, 1974). This literature review will focus on the latter, the conceptualization of bodegas and restaurants as part of a Puerto Rican natural support system.

Vazquez (1974, pp. 3-4), in a rare publication on bodegas, comments on the role of this institution in the community: "The bodega is a convenient location serving as a 'hang-out,' an emergency loan source, a place to get easy credit, a check-cashing place, and a type of information center . . . a place where its customers could find recreation, vocational and guidance counseling, and often someone to assist them in filling out forms." Agins (1985, p. 13) reinforces the points made by Vazquez: "It is here that plantains and chorizo sausage, religious candles, and Spanish romances can be purchased, where easy credit is extended, where gossip is traded, and where neighborhood men gather to play dominoes or watch TV."

The multifaceted nature of bodegas, along with lack of accessibility to supermarkets (i.e., inadequate public transportation and the presence of Spanish-speaking staff) allows these institutions to charge customers anywhere from 35 to 40 percent more than comparable items in supermarkets (Agins, 1985; Howe, 1986; Vazquez, 1974).

It can be argued that these establishments are first and foremost businesses, with all the tensions and issues associated with for-profit enterprises; provision of social services, as a result, are simply part of a calculated business strategy to increase market share and have "happy and contented" customers who will not only return but also spread the word to others in the community. However, this line of argument is too narrow in scope and neglects the cultural context of many ethnic-owned businesses. Service, in the instance of Puerto Ricans, is holistic in nature with the community having expectations that go beyond the strict provision of products.

Bodegas provide at least seven important services that extend beyond provision of native food: (1) credit (Agins, 1985; Delgado and Humm-Delgado, 1982; Fitzpatrick, 1987; Vazquez, 1974); (2) banking—cashing of checks (Fitzpatrick, 1987; Howe, 1986);

(3) community-related news and information (Agins, 1985; Delgado and Humm-Delgado, 1982; Korrol, 1983; Terry, 1992; Vazquez, 1974); (4) counseling customers in distress (Agins, 1985; Howe, 1986; Rierden, 1992; Vazquez, 1974); (5) assistance in filling out or interpreting government forms (Agins, 1985; Howe, 1986; Vazquez, 1974); (6) information and referral to social service agencies (Delgado, 1982; Delgado and Humm-Delgado, 1982; Howe, 1986; Korrol, 1983; Vazquez, 1974); and (7) cultural connectedness to homeland (Gonzalez, 1992; Hernandez, 1994; Levine, 1990; Raynor, 1991; Rierden, 1992; Rohter, 1985 a,b; Vazquez, 1974).

DESCRIPTION OF SITE AND METHODOLOGY

This study was based in Holyoke, Massachusetts. The city is medium-sized with a population of approximately 44,000, of which 13,500 are Latino (31.1 percent); the Latino population, in turn, is primarily Puerto Rican with this group numbering 12,700 (93.5 percent of all Latinos) (Gaston Institute, 1992, 1994). The Puerto Rican community is very poor economically with 59.1 percent having an income level below the poverty rate (Gaston Institute, 1994). This community is relatively young with a median age of eighteen, approximately half that of the general population (Gaston Institute, 1992). The study was undertaken in a forty-block area of Holyoke (residential and commercial districts) with a high percentage of Puerto Rican establishments and residents; this area of the city is almost totally Puerto Rican, facilitating the operationalization of the study.

This study on grocery stores and restaurants was part of a broader research project that identified a variety of Puerto Rican institutions that are part of a natural support system (Delgado, pending publication, b; Delgado, pending review). It is important to add that this overall asset assessment was undertaken by a group of ten Puerto Rican adolescents (male and female); these interviewers, once trained on undertaking an asset assessment, identified the institutions and conducted the interviews.

The goals of this asset assessment were to: (1) identify social service provision in general, and alcohol and other drug-abuse services in particular, (2) identify factors that facilitate or hinder collaboration with natural support systems, and (3) develop an asset inventory within a defined geographical area.

This asset assessment entailed the utilization of two questionnaires both of which were written in Spanish and English (please see Appendix). The initial questionnaire (Asset Location Form) gathered data on the following:

1. name of institution,
2. address,
3. telephone number,
4. type of institution,
5. name of field staff member, and
6. comments/impressions/observations.

The second questionnaire (Asset Assessment Interview Form) gathered additional information on the following:

1. year established,
2. hours of operation,
3. days of the week open,
4. type of social services provided,
5. leadership role in the community, and
6. comments/observations of the interviewer.

The latter category specifically focused on the following: (a) level of cooperation with interview, (b) degree to which interviewee expressed importance of the establishment in community life, and (c) physical appearance of establishment. Unfortunately, the interviewer responses were too general to assist with the interpretation of the data.

FINDINGS

Organizational Characteristics

The typical food establishment in our study has been in existence approximately 4.6 years, with a range from 1 year (N = 2) to 20 years (N = 1). Restaurants and grocery stores had an average existence of 6.5 years and 2.3 years respectively. The majority of both types of businesses are relatively new to Holyoke; four restaurants had been open three years or less and two had been open ten and twenty years, yet the oldest grocery store had been open only four years. The average number of hours open per day was twelve, with grocery stores (as expected) operating for longer hours with thirteen, and restaurants being open eleven hours. The range was from the low of eight hours (restaurant) to a high of eighteen hours (grocery store); the majority of these establishments cluster around the ten- to thirteen-hour-per-day period.

In examining the total number of days open and days of the week in operation, there were minimal differences within and between the two types of institutions. Three restaurants and three grocery stores were open seven days a week. (See Table 4.1.)

The two oldest restaurants were open seven days per week ("A" and "E"); restaurant "D," however, although only in existence three years, was also open the entire week. Grocery stores, as already noted, have a tendency not only to be open longer hours, but more days as well. If a grocery store was not to be open seven days per week, Sunday would be the day it closed—similar to restaurants.

In summarizing the operational characteristics, Puerto Rican establishments are relatively young in existence, open six to seven days per week, and an average of twelve hours per day. These institutions do not differ dramatically from those reported in the literature, with the exception of the number of hours open per week for bodegas—the literature reports an average of 108 hours (approximately 15 hours per day) (Carmody, 1972). Only one grocery store ("L") was open longer with 126 hours per week. This grocery store, it should be noted, had been in operation one year and the inordinate number of hours may reflect the necessity and difficulty of establishing a new business.

Provision of Social Services/Community Leadership

The primary focus of this study was to identify the types and ranges of social services provided by these establishments. (This study, it should be noted, made no effort to evaluate the "quality" of service providers.) Overall, the average institution provided approximately 3 services (3.36); restaurants provided 3.6 and grocery stores 3.0. The study identified three services provided by at least two-thirds of the establishments (integration of the lonely, interpreter services, and community leadership). (See Table 4.2.)

TABLE 4.1. Summary of Descriptive Data

Institution	Years of Operation/Number of Hours Open Per Day	Days of the Week Open							Total Number of Days Open
		Mon	Tues	Weds	Thurs	Fri	Sat	Sun	
RESTAURANTS									
A	20 years 11 hours	X	X	X	X	X	X	X	7
B	1 year 12 hours	X	X	X	X	X	X		6
C	3 years 11 hours	X	X	X	X	X	X		6
D	3 years 13 hours	X	X	X	X	X	X	X	7
E	2 years 8 hours	X	X	X	X	X	X		6
F	10 years 11 hours	X	X	X	X	X	X	X	7
GROCERY STORES									
G	No information provided								
H	2 years 12 hours	X	X	X	X	X	X	X	7
I	2 years 12½ hours	X	X	X	X	X	X	X	7
J	2½ years 11 hours	X	X	X	X	X	X		6
K	4 years 11 hours	X	X	X	X	X	X		6
L	1 year 18 hours	X	X	X	X	X	X	X	7

TABLE 4.2. Summary of Service Provision

TYPE OF SERVICE	REST							GROCERY STORE							Number of Inst. Offering Service
		A	B	C	D	E	F		G	H	I	J	K	L	
1. Credit		X					X							X	4
2. Information/Referral				X	X	X									3
3. Lonely Integration		X	X	X	X	X	X		X	X	X		X	X	10
4. Interpreter Services		X	X		X	X	X		X		X		X	X	8
5. Counseling						X									1
6. Food for the Hungry				X									X	X	3
7. Leadership		X			X	X	X		X	X	X				8
NUMBER OF SERVICES PER INSTITUTION		4	2	4	3	5	4		3	2	3	No Answer	3	4	X3.36

RESTAURANTS: X 3.6   GROCERY STORES: X 3.0

Integration of the lonely was mentioned by the most institutions (ten—five restaurants and five grocery stores). This service was operationalized to consist of some or all of the following: (1) individuals could spend time at the institution without having to purchase items or meals; (2) establishments could take telephone orders and deliver food for the frail and isolated; (3) customers could be invited to participate in events/activities and "festivales" sponsored or undertaken by the institutions—for example, customers (particularly men) could play dominoes; (4) customers had an opportunity to become connected to the community—staff would know the customer by name, family, etc., providing an option to become a part of a social network; and (5) these institutions provided customers with a setting and an opportunity to interact with other customers—one of the few settings where they would meet other Puerto Ricans in a friendly and respectful environment.

The above services highlight several key elements that categorize most Puerto Rican food establishments in the study. A customer is more than a customer; he or she has needs that go beyond nutrition. Second, an effort is made to personalize the service; a customer is first and foremost an individual, who happens to be purchasing a product or service. Third, a business, if it is to survive and thrive, must be an integral part of the community. Fourth, these institutions represent "spaces" in a community that allow Puerto Ricans to intersect. True, there are houses of worship that target Puerto Ricans. However, these tend to be small in size and a high percentage of the Puerto Rican community will not be a part of any one congregation (Delgado, pending review, b). Consequently, there are few public ("free") spaces in the city of Holyoke that foster this opportunity for contact.

The provision of interpreter services was mentioned by eight institutions (four restaurants and four grocery stores). This type of service was prominently mentioned in the literature (Agins, 1985; Howe, 1986; Korrol, 1983; Vazquez, 1974). Customers with limited English proficiency can obtain: (1) assistance in reading and interpreting "official" correspondence from government offices, (2) assistance in filling out forms, and (3) assistance from staff (on occasion) who will make telephone calls to government agencies and act as interpreters. This service is very essential in communities where English is not the primary language and social service agencies do not have sufficient numbers of bilingual/bicultural staff.

Community leadership was the third most frequently cited service by eight institutions (tied with interpreter services). Out of the eight institutions listing this service, five were restaurants and three were grocery stores. Community leadership could encompass any or all of the following: (1) sponsoring of community events and festivals, (2) making donations to other organizations that provide social services, (3) allowing the community to use space to conduct meetings (this is particularly the case with restaurants), (4) being a member on agency boards and advisory committees, (5) allowing community organizations to place posters or distribute information on services, and (6) allowing Puerto Rican candidates for local public office to distribute political material and meet with the community.

Surprisingly, only three institutions noted that credit was extended to customers (two restaurants and one grocery store). The literature on food establishments, particularly bodegas, notes the importance of provision of credit as a service. The availability of purchasing on credit has historically played a critical role in the lives of poor and working class people. Consequently, the "dropping" of this service may highlight the tension between "profit" and service to the community.

Three establishments (all restaurants) stated that they would provide information to customers concerning social services or make referrals to agencies, if needed. Three establishments (two grocery stores and one restaurant) provided food for the hungry—donating food to pantries or providing food/meals on the premises. Lastly, only one establishment (restaurant) provided counseling to those in need.

IMPLICATIONS FOR THE FIELD

The results of the asset assessment have raised a series of important questions pertaining to the role of food establishments within Puerto Rican natural support systems. The literature on bodegas highlighted a complex, highly evolved, and influential institution within the community. However, upon closer scrutiny, these institutions, with some exceptions, were not playing a very active service role within the Puerto Rican community, although they no doubt provide avenues for self-employment and employment of community residents, as highlighted in the literature (Burros, 1990; Carmody, 1972; Gonzalez, 1992; Hernandez, 1994; Levine, 1990; Raynor, 1991; Rierden, 1992; Rohter, 1985a, b; Sarason and Koberg, 1994; Stout, 1988; Vazquez, 1974). Unfortunately, the lack of literature on restaurants does not allow for a comparison; nevertheless, restaurants were not different from grocery stores in the nature and extent of service provision.

This cross-sectional study did not obtain data from an historical or developmental perspective. Consequently, these establishments may have started out providing a wide range of social services and over the years slowly stopped doing so; also, it may be that the findings are specific to one neighborhood in Holyoke and do not apply to the rest of the city or any other city in Massachusetts or the United States.

All of the Puerto Rican food establishments that consented to be a part of the study, however, did provide some form of social service to the community. Thus, food establishments do represent an avenue for possible collaboration with social service organizations. The nature and extent of these collaborative activities is dependent upon the following considerations: (1) the level of service provision and willingness of the food establishment to engage in collaboration; and (2) agency capability (bilingual/bicultural staffing), relationship with community (positive, negative, or neutral), and willingness to collaborate (Delgado, 1994).

Collaboration can cover a wide range of types of activities, with varying degrees of labor intensity and resources. The following case study of restaurant "E" serves as an excellent illustration of how collaboration can be planned and implemented and best typifies Evans and Boyte's (1986) conceptualization of community free spaces.

Restaurant "E" had been in existence three years, open six days per week and eight hours per day. Both owners of Restaurant "E" (husband and wife) are also foster parents to a number of children. In order to become foster parents, they have had to take workshops that have increased their helping knowledge and skills. Consequently, they have a basis from which to provide information and make referrals to social service agencies. The restaurant has several bulletin boards that provide agencies or community groups with the opportunity to post information of community interest and social services available within the community.

This institution has a contract with a local senior agency and provides space and hot meals for Puerto Rican/Latino seniors in the community. This space is also utilized for workshops, festivals, and recreational activities such as dominoes. This restaurant also sponsors or cosponsors recreational teams. Most Puerto Rican candidates for elective office use this setting to hold meetings, victory celebrations, and other events. Finally, this restaurant has an excellent reputation for generosity by providing food/meals to the hungry, and donating food and money for community events. The leadership role provided by the owners has also resulted in their participation on community agency boards, advisory committees, and task forces.

Not all institutions have the capability or willingness to undertake such active roles in the community. Consequently, collaboration may only entail the distribution of information on services or the posting of notices in food establishments. Puerto Rican grocery stores and restaurants can cosponsor community events or donate food, money, and space. These establishments can also provide community leaders for agency boards/advisory committees, as well as potential staff, as evidenced by the owners of restaurant "E" also being foster parents.

CONCLUSION

It is of great importance for the field of social work to continue moving toward an asset model in reaching out to communities of color; this model must also seek to develop community resources in addition to utilizing indigenous resources whenever possible. This article has provided a perspective on assets, namely the utilization of food establishments as part of a natural support system. Social agencies seeking to serve Puerto Rican communities with culture-specific services must incorporate natural support systems in planning and delivery. To be successful, however, these organizations must endeavor to plan *with* and not *for* the community.

Social agencies wishing to collaborate with Puerto Rican food establishments must become keenly aware of the challenges they will face. These challenges are far more complex than those encountered when seeking to collaborate with other social service organizations; natural support systems do not subscribe to the same set of operational principles and may not trust agencies. These establishments (a) do not utilize a "means test" to determine who is "worthy" or "unworthy" for services; (b) do not subscribe to the concept of catchment area and thus serve any person regardless of where they live; (c) do not undertake elaborate intakes or ask very "personal" questions; and (d) are very accessible geographically and hours/days of operation (many are open seven days per week and at least twelve hours per day).

However, as indicated in the case example, collaboration offers much promise and rewards for those organizations possessing the will to invest time and resources. These organizations must also be prepared to change the manner in which they view and engage the community; they can no longer take a deficit perspective on natural/ indigenous institutions. The free spaces/urban sanctuaries represented by Puerto Rican food establishments are not unique to this community; oppressed and undervalued communities across the United States, too, have their own natural resources.

APPENDIX

ASSET LOCATION FORM

I. Name of Institution/Nombre de Institución:

_____

_____

2. Address/Dirección: _____

_____

3. Telephone # / # de Teléfono: _____

4. Type of Institution/Tipo de Institución:

_____

_____

5. Comments/Comentarios: _____

_____

_____

_____

6. Name of Field Interviewers/Nombre de Entrevistadores:

_____

ASSET ASSESSMENT INTERVIEW FORM

I. **Background Information**

Información de Conocimientos

1. Name of Institution: _____

(Nombre de Institución)

2. Address: _____

(Dirección)

3. Telephone Number: _____

(Numero de Teléfono)

4. Name of Person Interviewed: _____

(Nombre de Persona Entrevistada)

5. Date of Interview: _____

(Fecha de Entrevista)

6. Year Established: _____

(Año Establecido)

7. Hours of Operation: _____

(Horas de Operación)

8. Days of the Week Open: _____

(Qué Días de la Semana Trabajan)

II. **Social Services Provided**
(Tipo de Servicios Sociales Ofrecido)

1. How do they help the community? _____
(¿Cómo ayudan a la comunidad?)

2. Do they provide financial help/loans? _____
(¿Proveen ayuda financiera/préstamos?)

3. Do they provide information on social services? _____
(¿Proveen información en servicios sociales?)

4. Do they provide friendship for lonely people? _____
(¿Proveen amistad a personas solitarias?)

5. Do they provide child care? _____
(¿Proveen cuido de niños?)

6. Do they provide interpreting help for those who cannot speak English?
(¿Proveen ayuda de interpretes para los que no hablan Inglés?)

_____

7. Do they provide advice/counseling? _____
(¿Proveen consejo/consejería?)

8. Do they provide housing/food for those in need? _____
(¿Proveen albergue/comida para los necesitados?)

9. Do they provide leadership in the community? _____
(¿Proveen liderazgo a la comunidad?)

10. Comments/Observations:
(Comentario/Observaciones:) _____

_____

_____

_____

Chapter 5

Puerto Rican Elders and Botanical Shops: A Community Resource or Liability?

INTRODUCTION

The professional literature points out that the health and social needs of Puerto Rican elders residing in the United States make this population at risk for a variety of social ills (Mahard, 1989); at the same time, Puerto Rican and other Latino elders face numerous obstacles in receiving services that are culture-specific (Espino, 1993). Consequently, the profession of social work and the field of human services must endeavor to develop innovative service delivery approaches to serve this population.

The development of a collaborative relationship between social agencies and Puerto Rican natural support systems is one approach with a high potential for maximizing limited resources (Delgado, 1994, 1995). Botanical shops (cultural variations of pharmacies) are a natural support system heavily patronized by elders, with the use of herbal medicine having a rich tradition within the Puerto Rican culture (Fetherston, 1992; Fisch, 1968; Harwood, 1977; Montana, 1991; Spencer-Molloy, 1994; Valdes, 1994). However, the professional literature has generally ignored this invaluable cultural/community resource for helping elders.

The author wishes to acknowledge and thank the key informants who were so generous of their time and Dr. Sharon Tennsdelt for her review and comment on an earlier draft of this chapter.

This project was funded through a National Institute on Aging Grant (AG 11171).

This chapter was previously published in *Social Work in Health Care*, Volume 23(1) 1996.

This chapter reports on a literature review and the results of a key informant survey of experts on the topic of botanical shops and how this resource can be utilized to reach Puerto Rican elders residing in the United States.

OVERVIEW OF THE LITERATURE

This literature review is divided into three sections: (1) definition and types of Puerto Rican natural support systems; (2) natural support systems and Puerto Rican elders; and (3) key themes related to botanical shops. These sections provide a broad overview of natural support systems and elders and set a context for examining key informant responses on the topic of botanical shops.

1. *Definition and types of Puerto Rican natural support systems:* The following definition of Puerto Rican elder natural support systems is based upon a composite of key themes noted in a key informant of survey social work scholars in Puerto Rico and the United States (Delgado, pending publication a):

> Puerto Rican elder natural support systems are a network of individuals, with or without institutional affiliation (family/ friends, religious groups, folk healers, and community institutions). They provide assistance (instrumental, informational, and expressive) on an everyday basis, as well as in times of crisis, and represent a community's capacity to help itself. Natural support systems also serve as a mechanism for helping Puerto Ricans maintain their cultural heritage. These support systems are accessible (logistically, psychologically, conceptually, and geographically) to all sectors of the community; the assistance provided originates from relationships (familial as well as nonfamilial) that extend beyond the provision of services, but also entail feelings of love, affection, respect, trust, loyalty, and mutuality. In short, natural support systems have responsibility for both giving and receiving assistance.

This definition of Puerto Rican elder natural support systems highlights both the extent, complexity, and importance of this resource in the lives of elders. In addition, the definition raises the importance of how resources are conceptualized within a community—natural as well as formal. Consequently, it is necessary to be very cognizant of how natural support systems get operationalized in a community; not all communities will have the same configuration of support systems!

Delgado and Humm-Delgado (1982), in their categorization of natural support systems, list four major overarching types: (1) family/friends and key neighbors, (2) religion, (3) folk healers, and (4) merchant/social clubs. Botanical shops fall into the last category. Merchant establishments are for-profit businesses that are community-based; these institutions are usually staffed, patronized, and owned by community residents. Merchant establishments, in turn, fulfill a variety of key roles that go beyond the selling of merchandise or services.

2. *Natural support systems and Puerto Rican elders:* The literature on the topic of natural support systems and elders is very limited in quantity and scope. Sánchez-Ayéndez's (1988) study of Puerto Rican elder women in the United States noted that children, husbands, friends, and neighbors provided a very reliable source of support during everyday life and crises (instrumental and expressive support). More specifically, daughters were the most reliable support even when an older husband was present (Sánchez-Ayéndez, 1992); however, elder women, too, provided support to those in their family network.

Cruz-Lopez and Pearson (1985), based upon their study in Puerto Rico, concluded that elders perceived their support needs as "generally" well met by informal (natural) support systems; these systems most likely consisted of family and close friends. Their findings were similar to those of Sánchez-Ayéndez (1988, 1992), even though their study was based in Puerto Rico, suggesting a continued presence of natural supports despite migration and acculturation.

Sánchez's research (1987) approached elder natural support systems from that of the caregiver and reported on the effectiveness of a training program for caregivers. This program provided natural support systems (relatives, friends, close neighbors) with information and support through a self-help approach. The author concluded that it is essential to provide assistance to the elder and his or her support system. Sánchez's study (1990) of Puerto Rican widows sixty years of age and older concluded that the adjustment to widowhood and the needs that arise out of this role are greatly facilitated if there is an active and supportive system of informal services provided by family and other significant individuals.

Delgado (1982) analyzed the role and extent of natural support systems in the lives of elders. However, he approached the topic from an elder perspective—namely, elders playing natural support system roles. Delgado concluded that natural support systems have a cultural base and are deeply rooted in history; thus, elders are instrumental in carrying on this tradition of helping. The concepts of mutuality and obligation are central to a Puerto Rican elder's conceptualization of natural support systems (Delgado, pending publication a).

Recent research (Gallagher, 1994) has highlighted the role of elders as providers of assistance, continuing a lifelong process of helping. Helfound (1994) comments on the role of elders as healers: "Many . . . who cannot speak English or afford frequent visits to the doctor, find an alternative source of care in trusted elders known for their home-grown herbs and celestial ties. People unaccustomed to fortress-like hospitals find comfort among these word-of-mouth shamans who can speak their language and fathom their demons" (p. 6). This helper role, as already noted, is also evident among Puerto Rican elders.

3. *Key themes related to botanical shops:* Botanical shops have not received an in-depth and systematic examination in the literature. The earliest and most comprehensive scholarly article on this subject was written by Fisch (1968), almost twenty-five years ago. Fisch's research was instrumental in highlighting the role of botanical shops in addressing health and social needs of Puerto Ricans in New York City. Borrello and Mathias (1977) not only described various aspects of botanical shops and folk healing, but also provided vivid photographs of this establishment.

Delgado (1979) and Harwood (1977, 1981) comment on botanical shops in their analyses of Puerto Rican folk beliefs and herbal medicines. Delgado (1979) developed a typology for classifying botanical shops: "These establishments can be classified into three types, depending on the extent to which they sell commercial products. Commercial botanicas are the most popular and common in the Puerto Rican community; in addition to providing some of the most commonly used herbs, they also sell a variety of more earthly items such as tickets to local dances, statues, and prayer books" (p. 36).

Fetherston (1992) provides an excellent description of what Delgado (1979) calls a "commercial" botanical shop:

> Santos Variety is a slightly misleading name for the store, since the variety is confined to four groups of products; the greeting cards in Spanish and English on the rack at the center of the sales floor, the music on cassettes in the center case, the cotton crocheted yarn in a rack at the back, and the paraphernalia of Santeria that lines the walls and dominates the scene. This concentration is duly noted on the front window, upon which is painted, in cheery yellow and red paint, the word, "Botanica." (p. 33)

Helfound's description of a botanical shop in Long Beach, California, compares favorably with Fetherston's description of a New York-based botanical shop:

> . . . Botanica Andio de Oro in Bell, offers a variety of religious articles to help the sick. . . . An entire wall is filled with brightly colored candles that feature pictures of saints said to protect against enemies and death. Oils to attract love or bring success in business are displayed in a cabinet across from a tiered altar with icons of saints, the Virgin Mary, and Jesus. (p. 6)

Delgado (1979) also describes two other types of botanical shops; "commercial-orthodox" types offer some commercial products, but also provide a wide assortment of difficult-to-obtain herbs. These shops also make referrals to local healers or have healers working on the premises. "Orthodox" botanical shops, in turn, are less common and serve a distributive role among "commercial" and "commercial-orthodox" establishments. Their only business is providing herbs and other healing paraphernalia and, like their orthodox-commercial counterparts, either make referrals or employ local healers.

Harwood (1977, 1981) addresses botanical shops from a cultural context of healing and healer; these institutions are an active and vital part of an extensive healing network within the community. These establishments not only serve as a focal point for obtaining herbal medicine, but also serve as a referral source for healers, as indicated by Delgado (1979).

In essence, the literature on botanical shops is in great need of updating based upon the dramatic changes in demographics and the potential impact of acculturation on Puerto Rican communities; in addition, these institutions need to be more closely examined with regard to specific age groups and the multifaceted roles they play in the community.

DESCRIPTION OF METHODOLOGY

The key informant survey is a substudy of a broader research project based in Springfield, Massachusetts. One of the aims of the parent study is to identify and describe current needs of African-American, Puerto Rican, and white, non-Puerto Rican elders. The study focuses on community-based long-term care assistance, receipt of informal care (natural support systems), and the use of formal services.

The goals of the key informant survey were fivefold: (1) develop a consensus and operational definition of botanical shops that reflects the current scholarly assessment of this support system; (2) identify what factors facilitate or hinder the use of these establishments in collaboration; (3) identify key services provided by these institutions; (4) develop a more in-depth understanding of how these establishments meet the specific needs of elders; and (5) elicit recommendations for how best to view and engage these community-based institutions.

In winter 1994, six Puerto Rican (five social work and one psychology) scholars were contacted by telephone and asked to participate in this survey. These informants were selected based upon a review of the literature and recommendations solicited from key Puerto Rican scholars in the field of human services in Puerto Rico and the United States. Although not all of these respondents were currently addressing the needs of Puerto Ricans, all had extensive work and research experience with this population.

The respondents were based at the following sites: (1) a western university school of social work in a large urban area (public); (2) an eastern university school of social work in a midsized urban area (public); (3) a southwestern school of social work in a midsized urban area (public); (4) a New England community-based Latino social agency in a midsized urban area; (5) a New England school of social work in a large urban area (public); and (6) a Puerto Rico department of psychology in a midsized urban area (public). Respondents represented a total of five states and Puerto Rico.

KEY INFORMANT RESPONSES

Respondents were asked to comment on various aspects of botanical shops. This section will summarize the responses and provide direct quotes whenever possible to highlight significant points.

1. *Consensus definition of botanical shops:* The following definition of botanical shops was developed based upon the input of all the key informant respondents and integrates the key elements they highlighted: Botanicas (botanical shops) are community-based establishments with an extensive history of meeting a variety of community informational, expressive, and instrumental needs in the physical, spiritual, and religious world within a Puerto Rican cultural context. These storefront institutions represent outlets for important Puerto Rican cultural traditions pertaining to healing/spirituality and are places where customers can socialize with others who share similar beliefs; in addition, botanicas represent opportunities for ownership of small businesses and employment for community residents. Last, botanicas do not exist in isolation from other Puerto Rican natural support systems, and as a result are integrally linked to folk healing and religion (spiritism and Santeria).

The previous definition places botanical shops as central institutions in the Puerto Rican community; further, the definition highlights the multifaceted helper role played by this establishment—religious, social, health, and transmitter of cultural traditions.

2. *Operationalization of Puerto Rican botanical shops:* This section examines the various elements that are present in botanical shops and why these establishments are generally so well regarded by the community; these institutions are complex in design and rich in cultural history.

Botanical shops provide consultation to elders regarding physical or emotional problems. One respondent noted the following: "The botanical shop owner is knowledgeable about healing qualities of herbs and other remedies sold in the shop. Knowledge of disease entities is also expected . . . frequently he or she may be considered a 'healer.' " It should be noted that the separation of physical and spiritual world problems is possible; botanical shop staff are prepared to advise and treat elders in both realms. Another key informant touched on this aspect: "Customers seek consultation of the spiritual world for addressing problems in the material arena (e.g., health and/or mental health, etc.)." However, the physical causes of health problems may entail referral to a health center/hospital; emotional/interpersonal problems, on the other hand, are generally addressed within this establishment.

Puerto Rican elders have very likely been exposed to folk belief systems as they were growing up in the culture and therefore are at greater ease in utilizing botanical shops. Although there is generally a great fear of the unknown, folk healing practices have been a part of the culture since the Taino indians inhabited Puerto Rico. Puerto Rican elders are "more likely to have been exposed to this already while growing up; this makes it much easier to see the utility of a botanica." These belief systems have also been influenced by African (Yoruba and Bantu) and Spanish conquerors/settlers (Harwood, 1977, 1981). Consequently, the belief that earthly events and conditions can be influenced by the metaphysical, i.e., spirits, has a rich history within the culture. Botanical shops, as a result, are institutions that can be considered medical/social as well as religious—a powerful combination.

As noted by Delgado (1979), folk healing medicines are action-oriented, and this further enhances the "effectiveness" and attractiveness of this approach:

> Herbs can rarely achieve therapeutic results without an elaborate process of preparation . . . usually involving several major tasks such as locating the right herb and preparing it to achieve maximum benefit by soaking, peeling, or heating it. These tasks can take anywhere from a few hours to several weeks to complete successfully . . . In addition to actively seeking a particular herb, which can entail visiting several botanical shops, the preparation process may require several stages. (p. 35)

This healing process requires an understanding of herbs and folk healing, along with a tremendous level of trust.

Botanical shops may also sell other types of healing/religious artifacts. One respondent stated: "Botanical shops in the last twenty to thirty years have become more diversified in selling other over-the-counter remedies (i.e., aspirins, cough syrups, etc.)." In the religious realm, "these institutions can sell candles, statues of saints, prayer books, etc."

These institutions are often very active in the community and help sponsor important festivals and sporting events, play leadership roles, allow the distribution of pamphlets describing community events, and provide a wide range of social services.

These establishments do not operate within the traditional logistical boundaries normally associated with social agencies (Delgado, 1994, 1995). Botanical shops are generally open seven days per week, twelve to fourteen hours per day. Hours and days of operation combined with centrality of location, and no paperwork to fill out on consumers, increases accessibility to the community.

3. *Factors that facilitate use of botanical shops:* Respondents were asked to provide reasons why botanical shops are popular within Puerto Rican communities and with elders in particular. Their responses covered six dimensions that ranged from accessibility to historical/cultural reasons.

Botanical shops sell products and services that have significant cultural meaning and history. As already noted, healing takes place within a cultural context with a particularistic set of meanings and expectations. Thus, various herbs and healing practices can be traced back historically and possess a prodigious degree of symbolism for Puerto Rican elders.

It is important to stress that the personal qualities (honesty and knowledge) of the owner and staff are essential for a botanical shop to survive economically within the community; a botanical shop that has a reputation for dishonesty will quickly have to shut its doors because the community will not support it.

Shops are located within the community and represent accessibility—not just geographical but also cultural and logistical. "Shops are invariably located in a barrio or neighborhood in which most, if not all, the residents are Puerto Rican (Latino)." Botanical shops are staffed by individuals who not only speak the same language as the customer, but are also very knowledgeable about community issues and needs. Invariably, owners and healers are also elders, further facilitating communication between customer and provider.

Botanical shops grant credit to customers who cannot afford to pay for various herbs and healing paraphernalia; this has the advantage of helping customers when they are in greatest need. However, there are undoubtedly situations where customers have not paid past debts and cannot return for assistance until the debt is cleared.

Botanical shops are part of an extensive social network. These establishments, as a result, do not exist in isolation from each other, or healing centers (spiritism or Santeria), or other natural supports: "These shops are a large part of the 'informal' network of our community, and as such act as a major mode of communication for reaching people. They help gain access to the elderly in need, disseminate information, etc." This relationship further enhances the degree of influence wielded by these institutions. Botanical shops make referrals to these centers and obtain consultation if needed; many of these shops are either owned by healers or employ healers to assist customers.

4. *Factors hindering collaboration with botanical shops:* All of the respondents noted that collaboration between social agencies and botanical shops must be based upon a series of considerations; botanical shops, in other words, are not without flaws, just as social service agencies are not perfect.

All of the respondents noted that not all Puerto Rican elders believe in using the services of a botanical shop. The following quotes summarize the sentiments of the key informants: "Some elders believe that the proprietor is working with 'evil' intents"; "I believe better-educated, middle-class elderly may not use botanical shops as frequently as lower-class (poor) elderly persons. However, middle-class elderly also use herbs and other botanical remedies"; "Elders who are 'overly Catholic' and fundamentalist Protestants"; "Elders who consider that botanicas are places for evil things. Pentecostal elders, for example, may not like to visit a botanica"; consequently, the degree of belief is a critical variable in the help-seeking process.

The key respondents, although not directly stating it, have raised issues concerning the "marginal" status of those individuals who patronize botanicas; these patrons are not only misunderstood by social agencies but may also be misunderstood by the Puerto Rican community itself.

Respondents raised the role of assimilation in this society as a key variable in diminishing the influence of botanical shops. One respondent noted: "I do see their role in getting information out to the elderly . . . and in this regard I do think social services should try to form good relationships with them. The twist, however, is that in forging these ties we may inadvertently be facilitating the demise of the botanica. In the end I do think that modern social services are basically competitive with botanicas, and if the idea is to protect botanicas, then maybe they should continue to exist at the edges of the social services." The development of a closer collaborative relationship with botanicas can serve to undermine the manner in which they conduct business and must be seriously considered by both parties. Customers, for example, may no longer depend exclusively on botanicas for most, if not all, of their medical care. Social agencies, in turn, may seek a more active role in dictating how a botanica prescribes medicines, particularly in those instances where herbal medicine can be considered harmful.

Another key informant stated: "Those most acculturated and assimilated to U.S.A. ways and those most educated are not likely to practice and patronize botanical shops." This key informant response does not bode well for the future of this natural support system. Although not all of a botanical shop's customers are elders, there is general agreement among key informants that most are elders. The passing on of elder customers without significant replacements from younger generations will result in a decreasing "market" for services. In addition, and equally as important, a diminishing number of Puerto Ricans will not enter the business, resulting in the likelihood of an important knowledge base of folk healing and system of care being lost to future generations. In essence, the significance of a major Puerto Rican healing institution will be greatly diminished.

One respondent specifically mentioned a concern that not all folk medicines prescribed in a botanical shop are healthy (Spencer-

Molloy, 1994): "Patients and shop owners need to be educated/informed about the potential interacting and negative effects of using herbs and remedies simultaneously with prescribed drugs." Not all herbs and remedies are unhealthy. Thus, it is very important to have an in-depth understanding of folk medicines, their properties, and how they are prescribed. Conversely, botanical shop owners/staff may not agree with everything a social service provider may be doing with an elder; there is an element of "mutual distrust" that cannot be ignored in the development of collaborative projects.

It is important to acknowledge that botanical shops do not exist in "harmony" with each other; they may be in competition with each other for customers. Thus, a collaborative project involving one shop may prevent other shops from entering collaborative arrangements with an agency. In essence, "turf" issues are not restricted to formal organizations.

The development of collaborative activities between formal and natural support systems is very labor intensive and will require considerable time, effort, and trust, on the part of both parties. "Negative perceptions by agencies, doctors, nurses, and social workers see botanical remedies/herbs as ignorance and lack of sophistication on the part of clients." It should be kept in mind that these two systems do not have a long-standing relationship and do not share similar views of how "earthly" problems originate; in addition, they do not share the same language (Spanish and symptomatology) or intervention strategies. This, however, does not mean that collaboration is not possible; it does mean that the barriers to collaboration are not "typical" of what is usually found in the human service field.

5. *Implications/recommendations for practice:* The key informant responses for practice implications can best be conceptualized developmentally and involve three types of collaborative activities. Each stage of collaboration, in turn, builds upon the previous stage and represents additional challenges and rewards for both botanicas and social agencies. A developmental approach serves to ensure that both types of institutions are well prepared to engage in activities that will ultimately benefit the community.

It is important to note that botanical shops do not exist in isolation from other Puerto Rican natural support systems. Consequently, social agencies must be prepared to conceptualize this resource as part of a greater network, with implications for an entire community. Collaboration with botanical shops, in turn, may lead to involvement with other forms of natural support systems.

The following recommendations seek to help organizations better plan and implement collaborative projects with botanical shops. These recommendations, in turn, must take into consideration the capacity of the organization to reach out to the Puerto Rican community; it is assumed that they employ staff that are capable (linguistically and culturally) of communicating with botanical shop owners/staff. In addition, these agencies must have a history of positive relationships with the community since trust will play an influential role in negotiations between parties.

Stage One: Information/Knowledge/Skill Development

Botanical shops are excellent sources for distributing information concerning elder services. "The shop can be a link in the chain to educate patients and the community at large regarding health care, good health, and prevention." These institutions, as already noted, are based in the community and are in all likelihood staffed by community residents. Customers who are elders themselves or family caregivers can disseminate information to the community. Thus, their accessibility represents an outlet that should not be overlooked.

Botanical shops are excellent resources for helping providers to obtain a better understanding of the community; social/health organizations must orient new staff to the community and this must include visiting botanical shops. Agency resource directories must note the location of these establishments, telephone numbers, and contact persons.

Botanical shop staff can be enlisted to provide in-service training on a variety of topics—help-seeking patterns, use of herbal medicines, health beliefs, etc. Use of these individuals will also facilitate the development of more complex and demanding forms of collaboration (Delgado, 1994, 1995).

Key informant surveys and focus groups, etc., that are community based, should include individuals who work in botanical shops. These individuals are in an advantageous position of having contact with the community, particularly elders who do not feel comfortable in seeking services from human service organizations.

Stage Two: Provision of Consultation

The provision and utilization of consultation by both parties builds upon and provides a more in-depth acquisition of information and knowledge/skill development. This type of collaboration has very specific goals of helping the consumer/client as well as helping providers (botanical as well as agency) develop better methods of meeting community needs. Both parties can develop formalized agreements that specify how consultation will be obtained, i.e., contact person, hours of availability, nature of help, procedures for emergency service, basic information needed to help consumer/client, etc. In addition, this type of activity can involve periodically scheduled meetings to discuss healing (consultee-centered consultation).

Stage Three: Active Referral Systems

Botanical shops, as already noted, make referrals to various types of folk healers, depending upon the wishes and belief system of the consumer. If the situation warrants it, they will make referrals to health and social service centers. However, it is important to note that when an elder does seek these services, they will rarely mention that someone in a botanical shop made the referral. "Puerto Rican elders frequently use botanical shops in place of prescribed medicines or in conjunction with prescribed drugs." Consequently, this important information is lost in the help-seeking process. Human service organizations must develop proper intake and record-keeping procedures that capture informal efforts at seeking assistance (Delgado, pending publication b).

If a botanical shop has a close and trusting relationship with a mental health/social service center, a referral or consultation is possible (Pachter, 1994). However, this type of relationship is rare. When it does exist, the relationship invariably is personal between the botanical shop owner/staff and a staff member in a local agency; if the staff member leaves the organization, this type of collaboration ceases to exist. In fact, rarely will there be a job description that specifically states that collateral contacts with botanical shops is part of a job; commitment to this type of working relationship is personal rather than institutional. Procedures for accepting referrals from botanical shops must be developed and staff job descriptions changed to reflect this added responsibility.

CONCLUSION

The review of the literature and results of the key informant survey have identified the need for human service agencies and botanical shops to work together to meet Puerto Rican elder needs. This community resource has historically played an instrumental role in the lives of elders in Puerto Rico and the United States.

The engagement of this resource, however, is not without limitations and serious considerations. In addition, collaboration—although highly desirable and needed—is also very labor intensive and can result in significant sectors of the community resisting this working relationship, i.e., fundamentalist religious groups. Nevertheless, it is necessary to move forward and make every effort to bring about a meaningful relationship.

In essence, there really is no forum to which botanical shop personnel should not be invited in order to express their opinions and elicit their support. The recommendations made by the key informants range in difficulty/labor intensity from relatively easy (distribution of information) to quite complex (development of a referral and intake system). Nevertheless, collaboration between formal/natural parties must be conceptualized developmentally over an extended period of time to ensure success and meaningful utilization of resources (Delgado, 1994).

In conclusion, one respondent summarized implications for practice very well when stating the following: "In the first place, human service agencies should recognize and place botanical shops in the network of community resources; staff should know the owner well, use him or her as a source of information in the community. Shop owners should be invited to community meetings and address health care concerns."

Chapter 6

Hispanic Natural Support Systems and the AODA Field: A Developmental Framework for Collaboration

INTRODUCTION

The AODA (Alcohol and Other Drug Abuse) field has only recently been paying attention to the use of natural support systems in the planning and delivery of services to communities of color. The use of natural support systems by any racial or ethnic group is greatly influenced by its beliefs, history, and traditions about helping its members as opposed to assistance from outsiders, as well as by the lack of available resources in the larger society (Weber, 1982). The impact of AODA in the Hispanic community is well documented (Glick and Moore, 1990; Mayers, Kail, and Watts, 1992).

There is little doubt that services to people of color must be based upon their cultural background; these services, in turn, must, whenever possible, be delivered by staff of similar background. The concept of natural support systems represents a perspective on how to plan and deliver culture-specific intervention. However, collaboration between formal (AODA agency) and informal (natural sup-

The research this chapter is based upon was funded through a Professional Services Contract (Order No. 90MF36045801D), Office of Substance Abuse Prevention, Rockville, MD.

This chapter was previously published in *Journal of Multicultural Social Work*, Volume 3(2) 1994.

port system) must be examined within a developmental framework—each stage has its advantages and barriers. This chapter
examines the use of natural support systems by the Hispanic community. The material presented in this chapter is based upon data
gathered through three site visits to Office of Substance Abuse
Prevention (OSAP) demonstration projects across the United States
and in Puerto Rico.

OPERATIONAL DEFINITION OF HISPANIC NATURAL SUPPORT SYSTEMS

Before proceeding with reviewing the findings from the field, it
is essential to present an operational definition of Hispanic natural
support systems as a means of establishing a set of parameters on
this concept. The definition that follows represents a composite of
input from nine academic/practitioners in the field of AODA who
have substantial knowledge and experience in serving Hispanics:

> Hispanic natural systems are composed of a constellation of
> individuals who relate to you, although not necessarily to each
> other, on a familiar or even intimate basis. These individuals
> are an important basis for self-definition and identity formation,
> and can be accessed freely on a casual basis or for the purposes
> of meeting specific expressive and/or instrumental needs. The
> concept of natural support systems extends far beyond the exis-
> tence of mechanisms that can be utilized as support systems and
> includes the individuals that *comprise* the support system (i.e.,
> while a church has the potential to be utilized as a natural
> support system, its utility lies in the personality of its religious
> leader); consequently, support systems are only as good as the
> individuals (natural support providers) providing the assistance.
> Hispanic natural support systems involve extended family
> members (both related and nonrelated), neighbors, friends,
> healers, institutions (including religious and other indigenous
> types), local self-help groups, and community leaders.

This definition does an excellent job of capturing the multi-dimensional aspects associated with natural support systems in Hispanic
communities (Delgado, forthcoming).

RESEARCH METHODOLOGY

The findings of this report were obtained through visits to three Office of Substance Abuse Prevention (OSAP) demonstration projects specifically focused on reaching Hispanic youth who are at risk. These sites were carefully selected to reflect a range of settings, different Hispanic subgroups, and different geographical areas (please see Note 1 (Appendix 1) for description of sites).

The criteria for the OSAP site selection consisted of the following: (1) community focus of project; (2) Hispanic setting or project representing a major component of a non-Hispanic setting; (3) willingness of project directors to participate; (4) OSAP funding for all or part of the project; (5) geographical area with high concentration of one of the three Hispanic subgroups; and (6) some aspect of Hispanic natural support system in place or planned.

Attempts were made to develop guidelines for OSAP site visits based on information in the following areas: (1) Hispanic community description; (2) project and organizational description; (3) natural support systems utilization in project activities; and (4) on-site observations concerning staff approaches/issues related to collaborating with natural support systems (please see Note 2 [Appendix 2] for a copy of the questionnaire used in site visits).

LESSONS FROM THE FIELD

The material gathered through the site visits is organized and presented as follows: (1) significant factors setting the context for NSS involvement; (2) barriers to developing collaboration with hispanic natural support systems (NSS); (3) types of hispanic NSS that lend themselves to collaboration; (4) importance of organization, staff, and community support in establishing collaborative activities; (5) a developmental framework for collaboration; and (6) conclusion.

Significant Factors Setting the Context for NSS Involvement

The site-visit dimension of the study purposely selected geographical areas that had high concentrations of each Hispanic subgroup noted in the sample. However, the findings from the visits highlighted the complexity and ever-changing demographics of the

Hispanic community. The sites, as a result, can best be placed on a continuum of diversity within the Hispanic community with Gurabo, Puerto Rico, being the most homogeneous (Puerto Rican), and Miami, Florida, the most diverse (Nicaraguan, Dominican, Honduran, El Salvadorean, Panamanian, Puerto Rican, and Cuban); Richmond, California, falls into the middle of the continuum (predominantly Mexican but with an increasing presence of Central Americans). The demographic trends made the study of Mexicans and Cubans as Hispanic subgroups impossible. Nevertheless, two significant issues emerged with respect to Hispanic subgroups that must be taken into account in the development of programs that attempt to involve Hispanic NSS: (A) acculturation and (B) documented/undocumented status.

A. *Acculturation:* The process of acculturation was evident in all three sites, with all Hispanic subgroups. Acculturation was particularly highlighted in Gurabo, Puerto Rico, with Puerto Ricans born or raised in the continental United States and returning to Puerto Rico. Values such as independence versus cooperation and competition versus cooperation reflected a dramatic shift between parents and their children; fluency in written and spoken Spanish represented another dimension of acculturation and a significant division between the two generations. Ironically, the process of acculturation served to diminish distinctions between Hispanic subgroups in the California and Florida sites. Acculturation level may dictate who can benefit from NSS. Highly acculturated youth may not believe, trust, or feel comfortable with turning to indigenous systems of care. Low-acculturated parents, in contrast, may not seek or embrace formal services. Thus, level of acculturation is a key variable in any form of NSS involvement in service delivery.

B. *Documented/undocumented status:* The impact of resident status, too, could be placed on a continuum with Miami, Florida, having the greatest number of Hispanic subgroups, followed by Richmond, California, and Gurabo, Puerto Rico, the latter being at the far end of the continuum, with a minimal presence of undocumented program participants. The fact that Puerto Ricans are United States citizens presents a different challenge to service delivery compared with Hispanics who are in the United States with an undocumented status. The undocumented Hispanic faces a greater likelihood of having limited access to their NSS which very often have been left behind in their native countries. Their social network will also be severely limited, for fear of having immigration authorities locate and return them to their native land. Consequently, resident status serves to separate Hispanic subgroups. Different geographical areas of the United States will have different undocumented Hispanic subgroups. Thus, efforts to locate and engage the NSS of undocumented Hispanics will prove to be very difficult and labor intensive when compared with Puerto Ricans or documented Hispanics.

Barriers to Developing Collaboration with Hispanic NSS

Respondents in all three sites were in general agreement concerning the four key barriers that they have had to address in order to effectively engage Hispanic NSS. Similar to the information provided by questionnaire respondents, the barriers described in the following text are not insurmountable. However, interventions must be carefully planned and staff must exercise tremendous patience. The professional literature on interagency collaboration notes numerous factors that hinder cooperation (Delgado and Humm-Delgado, 1980; Gans and Horton, 1975; Kraus, 1984). In exploring collaboration between Hispanic NSS and formal, caregiving systems, additional barriers become apparent and must be taken into account in any kind of feasibility study.

Lack of Trust

Cooperation cannot exist without a foundation based on mutual trust (Lenrow and Burch, 1981). However, the level of trust between Hispanic natural support systems and most formal systems of substance abuse care is minimal at best, and nonexistent at worst (Delgado and Rodriguez-Andrew, 1991). Generally, formal service providers are either unaware of, or have limited knowledge of, the influence of culture on help-seeking behavior (Delgado and Humm-Delgado, 1992; Fitzpatrick, 1990; Rio, Santisteban, and Szapocznik, 1990). As a result, culturally appropriate behaviors and attitudes may be misinterpreted as resistance, hostility, pathology, ignorance, lack of sensitivity and appreciation of what the provider can offer, or distrust (Singer, Davison, and Yalin, 1987). Natural support system providers may also have a wide range of stereotypes and biases concerning formal systems, seriously undermining the development of trust that is essential in any cooperative venture.

Conceptual Underpinnings of Assessment and Intervention

The conceptualization of causation and intervention will very often represent the cornerstone of professionalism. Nevertheless, for example, when comparing the theoretical orientations of substance abuse counselors and folk healers, similarities and differences emerge. Substance abuse counselors may argue that folk healers do not have a conceptual base to their practice and have not incorporated scientific principles and methods into their intervention, nor do folk healers have a rational basis on which to plan and implement intervention (De La Cancela and Zavala-Martinez, 1983).

As noted by Singer and Borrero (1984), "Unbeknownst to family and alcoholism therapists, however, the utilization of systems-like thinking about alcoholism and a family approach to its treatment is not an entirely new phenomenon. . . . During the course of this research, it has been found that a family approach is integral to the treatment of alcoholism among the folk healers observed" (pp. 155-156). It can be argued that folk healers do use theories of disease causation, differential intervention planning, and they also prescribe medication as needed (Singer and Borrero, 1984).

The question of who can legitimately practice healing (credentials) presents another barrier and is influenced by the conceptual underpinnings of assessment and intervention. As noted by Froland, Pancoast, Chapman, and Kimboko (1981):

> Professionals and informal helpers are coming from two quite different understandings about how help is given. Professional helping is generally based on standards acquired through training and experience; knowledge and expertise are valued in establishing the credibility of the help provided. These standards may have little meaning for informal helpers, as their helping is based on informal personal relationships, shared

experiences, and altruism, and their credibility is determined by the norms of exchange within the network. (p. 61)

Thus, varying credentialing processes are in action. Efforts to close this gap require special consideration to issues and disparate points of view.

Levels of Knowledge of Each Other's Mission and Work

The lack of information and awareness pertaining to the types of services which formal and natural support systems provide serves as a key barrier in developing collaborative strategies. The sources of information pertaining to how an agency operates, e.g., types of services, eligibility criteria, etc., are generally common knowledge and can often be found in resource directories. Unfortunately, these resource directories rarely, if ever, list natural support systems such as grocery stores, or are read by natural support providers.

Conversely, natural support systems do not have formalized resource directories of other natural support systems or formal systems—referrals and information sharing are usually done by word of mouth. Referrals from natural support systems to substance abuse agencies and vice versa, are often determined by the experiences of the referral source with the other systems (namely, highly personalized and determined by personal relationships rather than institutional agreements). Information sharing between Hispanic natural support systems and agencies is further limited by language and cultural barriers.

Service Delivery Structure and Logistics

The structure and actual delivery of assistance by agencies and natural support systems differ substantially. In examining the structure of service delivery, one quickly realizes that natural support systems do not function on a 9 a.m. to 5 p.m., five-day-a-week schedule. Healers, for example, cannot turn away an individual seeking help; consequently, they function very much on a crisis basis, as well as with appointments (Delgado, 1986); grocery stores and botanical shops are often open seven days a week, sixteen hours per day. In addition, natural support systems are very often found within the geographical area where the clients live and are not bound by catchment areas.

Other examples of structural and logistical barriers pertain to intake procedures, types of payment, eligibility criteria, availability of bilingual-bicultural staff, etc. Accountability concerns influence the above factors. The use of governmental and private funds necessitates the development of standardized procedures to provide accountability. Natural support systems do not receive public or private funding for services; they rely on individual payments and contributions. Thus, record keeping is not necessary. Natural support systems are accountable to the Hispanic community. The community, in turn, regulates who practices by influencing referrals.

Types of Hispanic NSS That Lend Themselves to Collaboration

Site-specific experiences in establishing collaborative activities reflect much of what was noted in the mailed questionnaire phase of the study. All three sites noted extensive involvement of extended family members, friends, neighbors, and indigenous leaders. These individuals participated in a wide range of activities from providing transportation, outreach, information, foster care, English interpretation when needed, and assistance in carrying out counseling assignments. Staff also made reference to involving other aspects of Hispanic NSS such as churches, folk healers, and merchant and social clubs (coffee establishments, bakeries, pharmacies, etc.). Consequently, all three sites were involved in reaching out to NSS. As expected, efforts to involve Hispanic NSS were not always successful or achieved without great effort. Respondents noted that families that were very dysfunctional often were very isolated from neighbors and extended family which made it difficult, if not impossible, to engage NSS in providing any form of assistance. All three sites referred to the challenges that undocumented individuals present. They are very often in great need but cannot access conventional human services; they are also very suspicious of government and strangers. This is unquestionably one of the major barriers in engaging NSS in certain Hispanic communities. Last, respondents also noted that NSS move to follow populations, leaving behind communities in great need. Many Hispanics who have uprooted, have done so at great personal sacrifice—very often leaving their support systems back home. There was one instance in which fundamentalist churches were reaching Hispanics. These Hispanics had moved out of the community, but still returned to worship. The churches were located in the community, but were not serving community residents.

Importance of Organization, Staff, and Community Support in Establishing Collaborative Activities

All three sites endeavored to hire Hispanic staff, preferably of the same Hispanic subgroup being served. One site (Miami, Florida) could not achieve this goal because of the range of groups being served—various Caribbean and Central American subgroups. However, they acknowledged the importance of being sensitive to the cultural values of these groups. Consequently, they were in the process of requesting technical assistance (training) to increase their understanding of these subgroups. Site administrators were cognizant that staff needed to be sensitive and open to nontraditional approaches to service delivery in the hopes of engaging NSS. Staff, with some exceptions, noted that their professional training had not prepared them to identify and work with Hispanic NSS. This was viewed as a serious limitation in professional education. Their experiences in working with other staff, internal and external to their organization, highlighted a certain "mind-set" that did not value cultural strengths and instead viewed Hispanics from a "deficit" perspective, making engagement of NSS impossible. The discipline of social work stood out as particularly beneficial as a result of an emphasis on community. This orientation valued work in the community, even though NSS might not have been part of any courses, etc.

In turning to organization, no setting could point out any organizational policy that specifically mentioned NSS or the importance of engaging this resource. However, all three settings were multifaceted in their approach to service delivery, including outreach activities and components, making it easier for staff to leave their setting and venture out into homes, houses of worship, etc. This was viewed as particularly important since staff could all point to organizations that did not allow this form of practice—namely, staff did not leave their organizations. Nevertheless, staff noted that organizations must be willing to change the methods they use to gather data, i.e., intake forms, to include categories focused on NSS. They also mentioned that it is very important that new staff, trainees, etc., be provided with an opportunity to visit the communities they serve prior to formally beginning their counseling, etc. This would provide them with a rich context in which to view problems and design culturally appropriate interventions. All sites mentioned how OSAP had provided them with flexibility in designing interventions that stress community involvement and NSS. This flexibility, unfortunately, is not prevalent in the field of human services.

Finally, all sites noted the importance of the community accepting them and their agencies, if significant work in the prevention arena was to transpire. Clearly, community acceptance was viewed as essential to any effective form of intervention. Distrust of organizations would result in noncooperation and active resistance. Consequently, staff noted that work in overcoming suspicion was time-consuming and labor-intensive. Services needed to be phased-in gradually with active involvement of all sectors of the community. In short, just because the organization wishes to work with NSS is not enough. Organizations need to start where the community is— namely, they must determine what it is that the community wants and needs first, then there may be talk about other services/approaches.

A Developmental Framework for Collaboration

As is evident in Figure 6.1, it is essential to view collaboration with Hispanic natural support systems from a developmental perspective, with each phase representing opportunities and barriers: Phase I—assessment of Hispanic natural support systems; Phase II—identifying and mapping of natural support systems; Phase III—relationship building; and Phase IV—programming collaborative activities. Failure to follow a developmental approach will increase the likelihood of failure in reaching and engaging this important community resource.

Phase I: Assessment of Hispanic Natural Support Systems

A systematic gathering of information is needed concerning Hispanic natural support systems. Data gathering can be accomplished through an approach that focuses on key aspects of natural sup-

FIGURE 6.1. Developmental Framework for Collaboration with Hispanic NSS

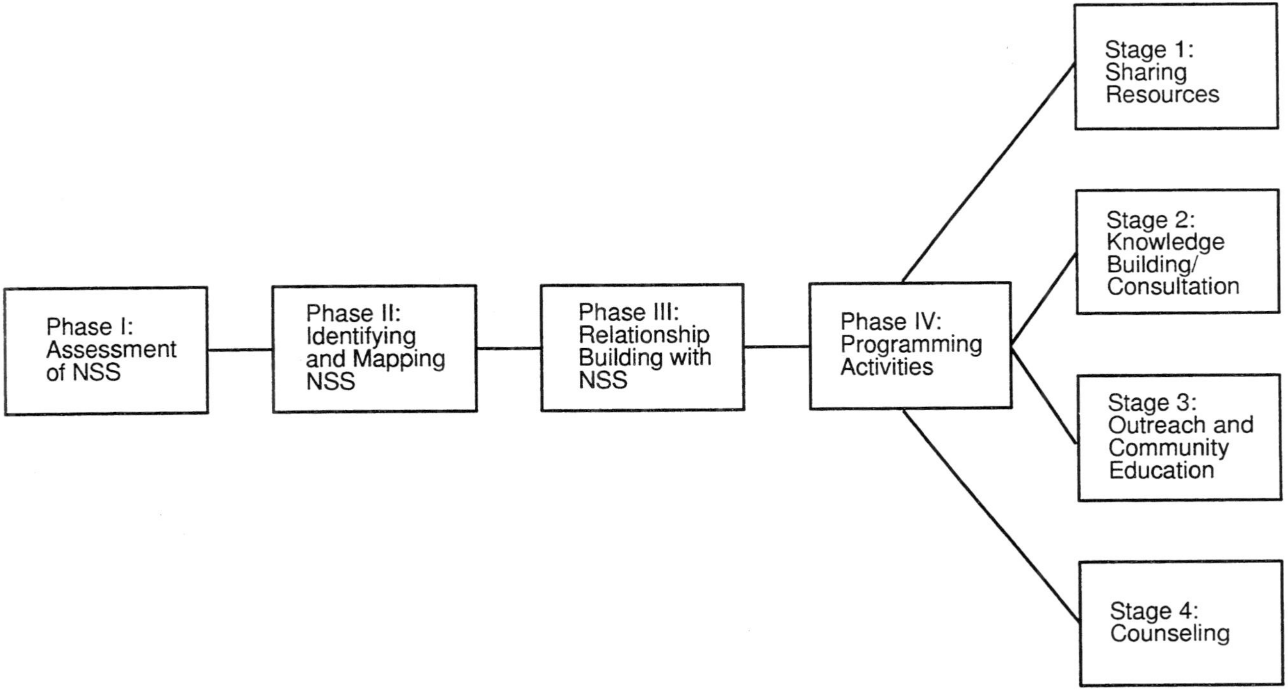

```
┌─────────────┐
│ Phase I:    │
│ Assessment  │
│ of NSS      │
└─────────────┘
       │
┌─────────────┐
│ Phase II:   │
│ Identifying │
│ and Mapping │
│ NSS         │
└─────────────┘
       │
┌─────────────┐
│ Phase III:  │
│ Relationship│
│ Building with│
│ NSS         │
└─────────────┘
       │
┌─────────────┐
│ Phase IV:   │
│ Programming │
│ Activities  │
└─────────────┘
```

Stage 1: Sharing Resources

Stage 2: Knowledge Building/ Consultation

Stage 3: Outreach and Community Education

Stage 4: Counseling

ports: (1) support system utilization patterns of past and present; (2) availability and capacity of support systems to meet current and future needs; and (3) potential of the system for collaborating with social workers.

In order to establish support system utilization patterns of past and present, the worker must determine what caused a client to seek formal assistance. Historically, what subsystem (e.g., family, healers, etc.) has the client relied upon? An added dimension that must be addressed is the frequency and nature of the client's contact with support systems. Does the client enjoy a balanced relationship with the support system? For example, does he or she interact with natural supports only when there is a problem, or do contacts transpire when life is going well, too? An example of imbalance would be the person who turns to religion during periods of crisis, but once the crisis is over, abandons this support system; or, the individual who, when in crisis, turns to certain family members, but is not heard from during periods of personal stability.

In assessing the availability and capacity of natural support systems, two crucial aspects must be addressed by staff: (1) client perceptions of the support staff's willingness and ability to assist, and (2) worker assessment of the system's ability to provide assistance. These two approaches are closely related, yet attempt to gather different types of information. Staff must endeavor not to rely solely on the client's perceptions and must, therefore, attempt to contact the support system in order to obtain a balanced perspective. Answers to such questions as frequency of contact, place of contacts, geographical proximity, type of assistance sought in the past, extent of mutuality, and characteristics of the support system provider (sex, age, etc.), help to provide further information on the extensiveness and availability of the support system.

The information gathered so far has focused primarily on the client and his or her support system, and is very instructive about a client's past and the nature of his or her coping behavior. Nevertheless, it does not provide information concerning the willingness of the support system to collaborate with the worker; consequently, the potential for collaboration must be addressed.

In exploring collaboration, four aspects need to be considered: (1) accessibility to the support system, logistically and psychologically; (2) worker's skills and knowledge (e.g., perceived trustworthiness, language abilities, knowledge of the culture and community); (3) the agency's willingness to involve itself with various types of natural support systems (e.g., philosophy, limitations placed upon staff, etc.); and (4) the client's willingness to facilitate/allow collaboration.

Phase II: Identifying and Mapping NSS

The process of identifying and mapping of Hispanic natural support systems is complex and labor-intensive. Unlike social networks which reflect a unique configuration of natural and formal support systems, natural support systems represent all potential sources of assistance. Information related to formal support systems is usually available in human service resource directories, to name a popular source of information. Natural support systems, conversely, are rarely listed in such directories or noted on agency intake forms, etc. Consequently, the identification and listing of natural support systems entails significant changes in how human service settings gather, list, and utilize data.

Delgado (1989) notes that agency intake processes must be changed to gather information on NSS. The intake process, including intake forms, represents a very important stage in substance abuse prevention. It very often represents the first "official" contact youth/families have with an agency and thus plays an important role in the relationship-building process. It allows youth/families and staff to explore expectations of what constitutes intervention, and it provides an excellent foundation for involving youth and their families in determining needs. Consequently, the intake process is the logical place to gather information on NSS.

Data on NSS must provide information on the following categories: (1) extent of NSS utilization prior to and while youth/families are receiving "formal" services; (2) gaps and duplication of NSS resources in the community; (3) location and accessibility of natural support providers; (4) characteristics of providers and those utilizing their services, i.e., age, gender, length of residence in community, etc.; and (5) trends related to the changing nature of NSS. Management information systems, as a result, must be able to provide data on NSS in assessing Hispanic community needs and resources. Once organizations make the necessary changes in data gathering, mapping of NSS can then take place.

Phase III: Relationship Building with Natural Support Systems

In order for staff to effectively interact with Hispanic natural support systems it is essential that they develop a relationship based on *confianza* (confidence/trust). *Confianza* expresses pure friendship, based on mutual understanding and appreciation, without obligation of kinship. As noted by Velez (1980):

> *Confianza en confianza* (trusting mutual trust) infers "trusting in the trustworthiness of self" by which mutuality is made possible. Without a firm sense of personal trustworthiness no commonality of trust can be extended or projected unto others. Trusting in the trustworthiness of others implies an ability to consider them trustworthy enough so that one will not need to be on guard against undesirable machinations on their part . . . Therefore at the individual level, *confianza en confianza* emerges as an important socially generated cultural value which functions to provide a behavioral map for self and others. (p. 46)

Valle (1980), further commenting on the importance of relationship in Hispanic natural support systems, notes:

> The natural networks extend ongoing contact with their linked members with the intent of assisting them to maintain their "heads above water" so to speak, utilizing culturally acceptable *confianza* building reciprocity approaches which permit the Hispanic in need to accept help with dignity and respect, allowing the maintenance of *orgullo* (pride) and the reduction of the possibility of *verguenza* (shame) due to an assumed dependency. Reciprocity and exchange dynamics are at the core of such interactions. (p. 42)

In essence, in order to develop *confianza*, staff must be prepared and willing to share of themselves and participate, whenever possible, in cultural activities within the community and the client's family. Staff may well be asked personal questions pertaining to place of birth, family background, and current marital status, and if appropriate, the number of children, their gender, and age.

This type of questioning will transpire when a client feels sufficiently comfortable with the worker. Thus, if the worker is going to ask numerous personal questions of the client in order to better know him or her, then the client may very well wish to reciprocate. It is not uncommon to hear of staff being invited to family celebrations (birthdays, weddings, baptisms, etc.) or community events. Failure of staff to share of him or herself will very often place a barrier in the client/worker relationship, severely limiting access to information and natural support system resources.

Confianza between worker and client develops over a relatively lengthy period of time and with considerable effort and personal involvement (Valle, 1980, 114-115). In addition, staff must have a sound understanding of the client's cultural milieu from an historical and theoretical perspective, as well as the current social-ecological environment (Valle, 1980, 113). Thus, staff will need to learn about Hispanic culture through self-study and actual visits into the community. Staff are encouraged to visit houses of worship, botanical shops, grocery stores, and social clubs. These institutions represent the most accessible point of entry into the community as a result of their visibility, cultural relevance, geographical location, and the nonstigmatizing nature of the service they provide—botanical shops may be exceptions. Staff may, once they are accepted by the community, use the above institutions as a community base to venture out to meet folk healers, for example. This process of information-sharing and relationship-building is both time consuming and very taxing since it may represent the very first attempt by staff to share and obtain information pertaining to Hispanic NSS. This process, however, can be facilitated if an Hispanic human service provider, or community leader (who must be well respected and liked by the community) can serve as a "bridge" between agency and community. Consequently, without self-study and knowledge obtained directly from the community, understanding of Hispanic NSS is not possible.

All phases of relationship building are greatly facilitated through use of Spanish. The use of Spanish is essential in attempting to involve all segments of a client's natural support system, even though the client may be bilingual. Consequently, staff, if not bilingual, can only communicate with those individuals who are English-speaking. Although interpreters can be used, the limited effectiveness of this method severely restricts information gathering and assessment.

Phase IV: Programming Collaborative Activities

The first three phases in the development of collaboration with Hispanic NSS can best be conceptualized as foundation development, with no actual service delivery involved. Implementation of these phases can dispel misconceptions and misinformation between clients and providers, which could thwart the development of any meaningful collaboration. Phase IV, in turn, explores joint-service delivery through sharing resources, knowledge building/ consultation, outreach and community education, and counseling. It is possible that collaboration may involve one or any of these stages; however, it is highly unlikely that the counseling stage can be developed without first attempting some of the other stages. The other stages, as it will be noted, represent activities that are not necessarily very labor-intensive or complex, but enriching to relationships prior to actual joint-service delivery counseling begins.

Stage 1: Sharing Resources. This type of collaboration was very common in all three sites that were visited. Sharing of resources can consist of a wide range of activities such as using space in a house of worship to hold group meetings with youth or to undertake training of parents; counseling is also possible if space is available and provides for a client's confidentiality. Agencies, in turn, can provide meeting space for community groups, if so requested. Indigenous institutions are invariably located within the community and are nonstigmatizing. However, as noted on one of the site visits, these institutions may be oversubscribed by agencies seeking space. For example, some houses of worship may find numerous organizations seeking space, making tremendous demands upon the setting. Some houses of worship may own transportation vans that can be used by staff in transporting youth to activities; agencies, too, may own transportation that can be used to help houses of worship in meeting the needs of their worshippers. Grocery stores may donate food or supplies for community-oriented events, etc. Sharing of resources is usually a good first step in the development of a solid working relationship because the commitment is time-limited and does not make excessive demands upon either party. In addition, it provides a good opportunity for both parties to "test" each other.

Stage 2: Knowledge Building/Consultation. This type of service can only transpire after both parties have a clear understanding of respective roles, strengths, goals, and a relationship based upon mutual trust and respect. However, this type of collaboration has prodigious potential in bringing formal and natural support systems together. Both groups can undertake formal efforts at upgrading knowledge and skills related to all aspects of the helping process. Staff, for example, can help ministers, folk healers, and leaders to recognize signs of substance abuse among the people they serve; Hispanic NSS providers, in turn, can help staff understand cultural factors that need to be taken into consideration in provision of substance abuse-prevention services. Consultation can be mutually given between Hispanic natural support providers and staff when requested. The professional literature on folk healer collaboration with mental health staff serves as an excellent example of this type of collaboration. Delgado (1979-1980) noted that consultation and training represented the most common form of folk healer utilization by mental health settings. Delgado (1979-1980) makes reference to five possible ways folk healers can be utilized in formal settings, two of which are training and consultation: "Type I involves the folk healer in a training capacity; he or she focuses on making presentations to professional groups. The frequency and nature of these presentations will vary from brief overviews of the cosmology governing earthly behavior to in-depth presentations of differential diagnosis and treatment . . . Type II affiliation also focuses on training; however, it differs by utilizing the consultation method of instruction. In this relationship, the healer can be called upon to provide case- or consultee-centered consultation for training purposes . . . " (p. 6). Delgado speculated that these forms of collaboration were the easiest to implement because they required minimal changes in agency structure/mission; the healer was involved for short time periods, and it represented an excellent way of involving the community without creating a major threat to agency personnel. These findings are well over ten years old and still very applicable today.

Stage 3: Outreach and Community Education. Collaborative activities focus on community outreach and education attempts to reach the greater community, unlike the previous forms of collaboration. Consequently, this stage of collaboration should entail activities that present a unified front to the community, are publicly placed, and have specific goals of reaching otherwise difficult-to-reach population subgroups. This form of collaboration would meet with minimal success if undertaken separately by each party. Collaboration activities can entail such actions as cosponsoring of community conferences/workshops, distributing information/materials related to substance abuse (grocery stores are excellent locations for posters and printed material for handouts), and getting assistance in reviewing and wording of information to make it more culturally relevant. Hispanic natural support providers can help agency efforts by "spreading the word" about programs and formally endorsing services. They can also accept and make referrals to staff. Delgado (1979-1980) mentions referrals as a form of collaboration: "Type III (folk healer/staff relationship) shifts the healer from trainer to referral agent. Through a formalized agreement, the healer is provided with a contact person within the . . . setting, and referral procedures from the healer and the . . . setting. Thus, the healer can both make and receive referrals" (p. 6). However, the type of collaboration outlined by Delgado requires a solid relationship between both parties and will entail close monitoring and follow-up to make sure that the client involved is satisfied. Needs assessments focused on substance abuse issues can be undertaken with active involvement of Hispanic NSS. Key informant approaches can and must involve Hispanic natural support providers (Delgado, 1982). Focused groups can also be undertaken tapping this community resource. In essence, Hispanic NSS must represent a significant aspect of any effort at assessing Hispanic community needs in the area of substance abuse (Humm-Delgado and Delgado, 1983, 1986).

Stage 4: Counseling. This stage of collaboration offers the greatest challenge to Hispanic natural support providers and staff. The sharing of a client between two or more parties is highly unusual in the counseling arena. Whittaker (1983) has outlined five possible strategies for helping, two of which do not involve collaboration between staff and natural support providers (staff helps client without involving NSS; NSS assists client without involving staff). However, three strategies attempt to "blend" these two systems together:

1. Social support network as a focus and locus for direct, face-to-face, professional interaction. Family network therapy and community network therapy represent two examples of this form of collaboration.
2. Social support network as supplement, complement, enhancement to professional helping. This may entail creating a support group for parents of children who are abusing drugs.
3. Social support network as primary method of help; professional helping ancillary—supportive. This could entail periodic treatment sessions with an individual member of a community self-help group. (pp. 56-57)

The framework developed by Whittaker serves as an excellent starting point from which to consider various types of collaboration between staff and Hispanic natural support providers. The type of relationship will be greatly influenced by a wide range of factors such as availability and willingness of natural supporters to get involved with professional staff, the depth of the relationship between both parties, organizational-community willingness to allow this type of work relationship, and funding considerations for the formal organization.

Nevertheless, this form of collaboration is very possible for programs that are based in the community and have a willingness to attempt such activities. There is a word of caution, however. The literature makes reference to various forms of collaboration involving counseling. However, if programs hope to utilize folk healers, it should be noted that past efforts at this form of collaboration have achieved mixed results (Singer and Borrero, 1984; Delgado, 1979-1980). Even though folk healers represent a significant natural support resource in the community, efforts at formally involving them can result in strong community opposition. Religious and community leaders may believe that folk healers work with the "devil" and should not be legitimized through formal working relationships with agencies; Hispanic providers may resist this effort because they may believe that use of folk healers represents a significant step backward for the community (De La Cancela and Zavala-Martinez, 1983); and last, the community may resist getting involved with projects that utilize folk healers for fear of how this would impact on their lives. Consequently, it is important that *all* aspects of a possible collaborative relationship be considered prior to efforts at formulating a working relationship.

CONCLUSION

This article has presented a developmental framework for establishing closer collaboration between Hispanic natural support systems and AODA agencies. This perspective is based on the premise that culture-specific intervention is necessary to reach a grossly underserved community. There is little question that collaboration between formal and informal spheres is very difficult, if not impossible, without careful preparation and staff willing and able to venture into the Hispanic community. Consequently, collaboration will be labor and time intensive. However, the rewards far outweigh the limitations!

APPENDIX 1

Note 1: Description of Sites

As already noted, these sites were carefully selected to reflect a range of settings, different Hispanic subgroups, different geographical areas, and settings:

Site 1—Miami, Florida (Year I). This project provides a multifaceted prevention/early intervention approach to Hispanic youth (ages 8 to 14) and their families. The City of Miami is highly urbanized and with rich diversity of ethnic groups. Hispanic subgroups are primarily represented by Cubans, Puerto Ricans, Nicaraguans, El Salvadorians, Dominicans, and Colombians; in addition, there is Hispanic representation from probably all Latin-American countries. The host organization provides a wide range of services to youth and their families covering all phases of intervention (prevention, early intervention, and treatment).

Site 2—Gurabo, Puerto Rico (Year I). This project seeks to reduce risk factors associated with substance abuse through implementation of a school-based curriculum. Efforts will also be made to involve a network of parents and community leaders in both learning and extracurricular activities. The population of children will be Puerto Rican (no other Hispanic subgroup is present) and elementary-school aged. The Puerto Rican Extension Service has a rich history of community-based service delivery and efforts to include a wide sector of the community in all aspects of service provision.

Site 3—Richmond, California (Year III). This project is located within a short commuting distance of San Francisco. It attempts to reduce the risk factors of elementary-aged children through provision of counseling and recreational services that are school-based, and comprehensive in nature, and foster development of positive family/community interactions. This project, unlike the two other projects visited, did not limit itself to Hispanics and attempted to reach other people of color. Both organizations have a long history of community involvement and collaborative efforts. Consequently, the thrust toward involving NSS was not alien and met with a positive response.

APPENDIX 2

Note 2: Questionnaire for Site Visits

*GUIDELINES FOR OSAP HISPANIC NATURAL SUPPORT SYSTEM
ON-SITE VISIT IDENTIFYING INFORMATION*

Name of respondent(s):

Agency name:

Address and telephone number:
Date of visit:

HISPANIC COMMUNITY DESCRIPTION
1. History of community in geographic area: _____
_____
_____
_____
_____

2. Key demographic characteristics: _____
_____
_____
_____

3. How has drug abuse been defined as a problem in the community?
_____
_____
_____
_____

PROJECT AND ORGANIZATIONAL DESCRIPTION
1. Project goals: _____
_____
_____
_____
_____

2. Target population: _____

_____

_____

_____

3. Method of intervention: _____

_____

_____

_____

4. High-risk indicators used in grant application: _____

_____

_____

_____

5. Mission/purpose of organization: _____

_____

_____

_____

6. Type of setting/range of services/collaboration mode: _____

_____

_____

_____

7. Agency policies of particular relevance to NSS: _____

_____

_____

_____

8. Staffing patterns and characteristics (gender, ethnicity, education, age, discipline): _____

_____

_____

_____

_____

9. Funding sources (how they facilitate or hinder use of NSS): ____

_____

_____

_____

_____

_____

NATURAL SUPPORT SYSTEMS

1. Types/functions/characteristics of key NSS providers: _____

_____

_____

_____

_____

_____

2. Any particular types of NSS lend themselves to use or non-use in prevention: _____

_____

_____

_____

_____

3. History of NSS systems in community: _____

_____

_____

_____

_____

_____

4. Issues and considerations in setting up activities involving NSS:

_____

_____

_____

_____

_____

_____

5. Any insurmountable obstacles that can be identified: _____

_____

_____

_____

_____

6. What process was used to establish joint activities with NSS?

_____

_____

_____

_____

7. Does the program have any materials that shed light on use/non-use of NSS? _____

_____

_____

_____

_____

8. Recommendations for OSAP and other funding sources: _____

_____

_____

_____

_____

_____

ON-SITE OBSERVATIONS
1. Role of personal relationships (individual served, provider): ___

_____

_____

_____

_____

_____

_____

2. Characteristics of staff using NSS: _____

_____

_____

_____

_____

_____

3. Agency policy or staff determined use of NSS: _____

_____

_____

_____

_____

4. Any particular sequencing of services/collaboration agreements:

_____

_____

_____

_____

_____

5. How widely accepted is the concept of NSS among staff, board, community? _____

_____

_____

_____

_____

6. Are there any activities that lend themselves to using NSS?

_____

_____

_____

7. How does use of NSS and the concept of empowerment relate?

_____

_____

_____

_____

_____

8. GENERAL COMMENTS AND OBSERVATIONS

_____

_____

_____

_____

_____

_____

_____

_____

_____

_____

Chapter 7

Hispanic Natural Support Systems and Alcohol and Other Drug Services: Challenges and Rewards for Practice

INTRODUCTION

The last decade has witnessed a dramatic increase in the number of Hispanics residing within the United States (Pinal and De Navas, 1990; Valdiveso and Davis, 1988); it is projected that the increases will continue into the twenty-first century (Hayes-Bautista, Schink, and Chapa, 1988). Consequently, issues confronting this population are of great interest throughout the United States. In this light, youth at risk among Hispanics comprise a population of considerable interest to the AODA field. The professional literature suggests that natural support systems (NSS) are an important ingredient of Hispanic culture and a key factor that should be integrated into all aspects of service delivery (Delgado and Humm-Delgado, 1982; De la Rosa, 1988; Valle and Bensussen, 1985; Valle and Vega, 1980).

Nevertheless, as noted by Delgado and Rodriguez-Andrew (1991) in their review of sixteen Office of Substance Abuse Prevention (OSAP) Hispanic grant applications including site visits to a majority of the programs: "In general, no site addressed Hispanic natural support systems in a planned and systematic fashion . . . the use of natural support systems has not been conceptualized as a valuable

The research this chapter is based upon was funded through a Professional Services Contract (Order No. 90MF36045801D), Office of Substance Abuse Prevention, Rockville, MD.

This chapter was previously published in *Alcoholism Treatment Quarterly*, Volume 12(1) 1995.

caregiving system; as a result, these systems have not been prioritized in the delivery of services to Hispanics" (p. 18). Thus, there exists a tremendous gap between practice and theory.

Further, the professional literature highlights that there is no single Hispanic culture. There are cultural differences among Mexican American, Puerto Rican American and Cuban American populations. This suggests that before one can generalize to an "Hispanic" population about a concept such as natural support systems, it is essential to examine this concept with respect to each of these cultural Hispanic subgroups.

The purpose of this chapter is to help AODA settings to better identify and utilize Hispanic natural support systems in their efforts to provide culture-specific services.

A LITERATURE OVERVIEW OF HISPANIC NSS AND SUBSTANCE ABUSE PREVENTION/INTERVENTION

The review did *not* attempt to locate and analyze all of the literature on natural support systems. It was felt that this task had been accomplished by various scholars and that it would detract from the primary purpose of this chapter.

This section will consist of four categories: (1) definitions of key concepts, (2) four substance abuse prevention perspectives on Hispanic natural support systems, (3) a framework for analyzing Hispanic natural support systems, and (4) strategies for establishing collaboration (lessons from the literature). The intent of this section is to provide a foundation for examining findings from a survey mailed to nine "experts" on this topic.

Definitions of Key Concepts

It is important to provide definitions of four concepts that form the cornerstone of this chapter: Hispanic natural support systems (NSS), natural support providers, and substance abuse. These concepts are quickly finding their way into the substance abuse field. However, they each have differing connotations to service providers. Although the term "Hispanic" is widely used in this society and among service providers, different definitions of who is an Hispanic are common; frequently used criteria are: country of origin, primary language, surname, country of origin of parents, location of birth, and self-disclosure (Humm-Delgado and Delgado, 1983). For our purposes, self-disclosure will be the definition that will be used.

Garbarino's (1983) research of the literature identified thirteen concepts of help or helper, many of which are used interchangeably (natural caregiving, self-help, neighborhood network consultant, support group, social network, formal and informal support system, helping network, natural helper, lay helper, central figure, natural helping network, social support network, and mutual aid); this abundance of concepts focused on "natural" helping very often leads to confusion. Consequently, this report will utilize Baker's (1977) definition of natural support systems as a baseline from which to examine Hispanic NSS:

> The word 'natural' is used to differentiate such systems from the professional care-giving systems of the community . . . Natural support systems include family and friendship groups, local informal care-giving professionals and mutual help groups. In most communities there exists a network of individuals and groups who band together to help each other in dealing with a variety of problems in living. Such groupings which provide attachments among individuals or between individuals and groups such that adaptive competence is improved in dealing with short-term crises and life transitions are referred . . . to as natural support systems. (p. 139)

The above definition provides a solid foundation that incorporates many of the concepts of help described by Garbarino (1983) and allows for examining of the role and importance of natural support systems in Hispanic communities.

Natural support providers represent the helpers found within natural support systems. These individuals, as it will be noted in other sections of the literature review, provide instrumental and expressive assistance, based upon the position they occupy within their respective systems (i.e., religious minister/priest not only helps with spiritual needs but may also provide a range of social services; a grocery store owner may sell food and other items, but may still provide credit and social contact, and make necessary referrals).

Consequently, the terms provider and systems may be used inter-changeably throughout this report.

Last, substance abuse refers to illicit and licit chemicals—the latter include cigarettes, alcohol, and prescription and over-the-counter me-dications (Newcomb and Bentler, 1988). These substances can be taken in various combinations and amounts. This chapter does not attempt to differentiate between substances or degrees of abuse.

Four Substance Abuse Service Perspectives on Natural Support Systems

Substance abuse programs can take one of four possible ap-proaches to natural support systems with each approach having far-reaching implications for the structure and provision of services to Hispanic communities (Delgado, 1995). One approach is to ig-nore natural support systems in all aspects of service delivery. Sim-ply, this will manifest itself by the provider/agency not asking an Hispanic client about his/her natural support systems and thus, not taking them into account in planning intervention. Unfortunately, this is probably the most common approach in substance abuse and other human service fields.

A second approach entails undermining natural support systems. When Hispanic clients volunteer information concerning key indi-viduals in their life or belief systems, the provider will actively try to change the client; for example, if a client believes that his/her problems may be the result of evil spirits, a provider may either downplay their significance or raise serious concerns about the client's mental state (De La Cancela and Zavala-Martinez, 1983; Singer, 1984; Singer and Borrero, 1984).

Turning to culturally sensitive approaches, substance abuse pro-viders can modify services to incorporate key cultural themes or collaborate with natural support systems. The former entails learn-ing about a client's cultural belief system and making every effort to modify intervention accordingly. For example, if the client defines family along extended lines, the provider may involve extended family members, neighbors, and friends in family counseling ses-sions. The latter approach is the most progressive and the central focus of this report, namely, agencies and providers working along-side natural support systems. Collaboration can occur in a variety of spheres: case finding, provision of transportation, use of community space, information dissemination, cotreatment, etc.

A Framework for Analyzing Hispanic Natural Support Systems

Hispanic natural support systems have received their share of attention in the professional substance abuse literature (Delgado, 1989; De La Rosa, 1988; Delgado and Rodriguez-Andrew, 1991; Rio, Santisteban, and Szapocznik, 1990). The literature identifies two basic approaches to operationalizing the concept of Hispanic NSS. Valle and Vega (1980), based upon their work with Mexican-Americans, have operationalized NSS as consisting of three significant subsystems: (1) aggregate (group membership) natural support networks, (2) linkperson (nongroup reciprocal relationships), and (3) kinship—familial, consanguineal, networks.

Delgado and Humm-Delgado (1982), based upon their work with Puerto Ricans, present a framework for analyzing natural support systems that takes a broader community perspective. Their framework consists of four major helping categories: (1) extended family (in addition to blood-related relatives, this category can include friends, neighbors, and significant others); (2) folk healers (spiritists, *santeros, santiguadores, curanderos,* and herbalists); (3) religion (Catholics, Pentecostals, Seventh-Day Adventists, and Jehovah's Witnesses); and (4) merchant and social clubs (e.g., grocery stores, botanical shops, market places, hometown clubs, and barber/beauty shops).

Thus, the reader can utilize either of these frameworks in helping to identify and study natural support systems within their communities. It is important to note that the above operationalizations reflect general categories and are not exhaustive in nature—namely, that depending upon the geographical and Hispanic community being addressed, other forms of natural supports may be present and need to be taken into account in service delivery.

Strategies for Establishing Collaboration (Lessons from the Literature)

It is important to establish key principles that should guide the collaboration between substance abuse programs and natural support systems. However, before doing this it is necessary to examine basic rationales for substance abuse agencies' developing collaboration with natural support systems: (1) cost effectiveness—more resources being provided and in a coordinated manner; (2) social participation of the community—natural support system providers are well-equipped to identify needs and make necessary referrals, and greater community participation means greater community acceptance of services; and (3) organizational effectiveness—natural support systems are culturally relevant, accessible, and can increase the capacity of an organization in reaching difficult-to-reach clients (Froland, Pancoast, Chapman and Kimboko, 1981). However, regardless of the reasons for developing collaborative efforts with natural support systems, substance abuse service providers must develop plans of action based upon a vision of what they hope to accomplish. This vision, in turn, translates into guiding principles.

The principles developed by Froland, Pancoast, Chapman, and Kimboko (1981) in the early 1980s are still very relevant today and represent an excellent starting point for substance abuse programs attempting to collaborate with Hispanic natural support systems. Substance abuse counselors must:

1. See clients as individuals with strengths and resources as well as problems and needs. This principle utilizes resiliency as opposed to deficits, as a basis for establishing a relationship.
2. Recognize the importance of an enduring network of social relationships. Substance abuse does not transpire within a social vacuum but in a social/cultural context involving multiple individuals. These individuals, in turn, must be taken into account in the assessment and planning of intervention.
3. Recognize that equality status should prevail between natural support providers and professionals. In effect, natural support providers should not be considered "paraprofessionals" because they may lack formal education or credentials.
4. Share responsibility of care. People in need should not be restricted, or made to feel guilty, for utilizing formal or informal resources. The lack of bilingual/bicultural providers will very often necessitate a broad approach to service provision—a team approach with each member meeting specific needs of the client.

5. Respect the way individuals and local groups define their problems. Solutions must be based upon the social reality of the client/ community. (pp. 167-168)

The above principles are only suggestions. Nevertheless, it is essential for AODA providers to have a clear set of guiding principles to help them develop collaboration strategies. Failure to do so will result in confusion, misdirected efforts, and limited impact on service needs of Hispanic clients.

A CONSENSUAL OPERATIONAL DEFINITION OF HISPANIC NSS

The following definition of Hispanic natural support systems represents a composite of input from respondents in the mailed questionnaire phase of this study: A total of nine academics/practitioners were selected for the second phase of the study. These individuals, in consultation with the OSAP project officer, were selected because of their expertise on natural support systems (conceptualization, experience with implementation, and their use in the development of substance abuse prevention strategies for high risk Hispanic youth). In addition, effort was made to ensure that adequate representation of Mexican, Puerto Rican and Cuban backgrounds were reflected in the sample.

Hispanic natural systems are composed of a constellation of individuals who relate to you, although not necessarily to each other, on a familiar or even intimate basis. These individuals are an important basis for self-definition and identity formation, and can be accessed freely on a casual basis or for the purposes of meeting specific expressive, and/or, instrumental needs. The concept of natural support systems extends far beyond the existence of mechanisms that can be utilized as support systems and includes the individuals that *comprise* the support system (e.g., while a church has the potential to be utilized as a natural support system, its utility lies in the personality of its religious leader); consequently, support systems are only as good as the individuals (natural support providers) providing the assistance. Hispanic natural support systems involve extended family members (both related and nonrelated), neighbors, friends, healers, institutions (including religious and other indigenous types), local self-help groups, and community leaders.

The above definition conveys the richness and complexity of Hispanic natural support systems; in fact, it is impossible to conceptualize Hispanic NSS without taking into account the community context in which it is located.

In examining in greater detail the conceptual underpinnings of the respondents' definition of natural support systems, five important themes emerge:

1. The importance of personal relationships in facilitating the help-seeking process. How well does the NSS provider relate to the person in need and the community? It is extremely important that the NSS provider have a reputation that is beyond question. This reputation must include competence, respectfulness, friendliness, and ability to maintain confidentiality. This finding is very consistent with the literature on Hispanic help seeking (Bernal and Flores-Ortiz, 1982). Gender must be taken into consideration in the help-seeking process, that is, males may display a higher degree of comfort dealing with males, and females with females.

2. NSS must be accessible geographically and psychologically. The fact that NSS are community-based is very important. However, they must also be psychologically accessible. Namely, the person seeking help must be able to expect respect, understanding, validation, and intervention that is culturally appropriate; in addition, help should be provided by someone of the same Hispanic subgroup. Thus, accessibility and personal relationships are closely integrated and necessary to Hispanic NSS.

3. Any definition of Hispanic NSS must take into account community leaders who represent the community to the larger society. These individuals may very well undertake causes that impact on many members of the community and thus meet a wide range of instrumental and expressive needs. In addition,

it is essential to incorporate self-help and mutual-aid groups that may be emerging within communities. This no doubt takes into account many twelve-step programs.

4. Hispanic NSS play an important role in helping to form and maintain one's identity as an "Hispanic" by providing role models, a sense of history, and the opportunity for the community to take care of its own within a cultural context that is rich in meaning and provides hope for the future.

5. Family must be central to any form of NSS. Family is defined in a broad manner to encompass blood relatives, relatives by marriage, close family friends, and special neighbors—the latter are often referred to as being "just like family."

WHAT HISPANIC NSS CONSIST OF, HOW THEY FUNCTION, AND HOW THEY CAN BE USED IN PREVENTION

This section will provide a cultural context from which to examine Hispanic NSS. In addition, issues and suggestions related to operationalizing the concept of Hispanic NSS for services will be delineated.

What do Hispanic NSS consist of? Family is central to any viable Hispanic natural support systems. Family members play an influential role in providing emotional support, assistance with ecological demands (advocacy, transportation, financial assistance), among other needs. In fact, family members may fulfill a variety of natural support provider roles in addition to usual family member roles. Folk healers, for example, may help strangers, but can also help family members. Family members, in turn, do not have to be folk healers to provide folk cures. In essence, family is the *core* of any form of natural support system.

Religion represents another important element of Hispanic NSS. Catholicism still plays an influential role within the community. However, various other religious groups such as Pentecostals and Seventh-Day Adventists are playing significant roles in addressing community substance abuse problems. Folk healers, representing a different aspect of spirituality, are an important community health resource. These healers are found in all of the Hispanic subgroups being addressed in this study, with each group having specific healers (Delgado and Humm-Delgado, 1982). Last, merchant and social clubs were mentioned by four respondents. One respondent noted that this NSS had experienced diminished influence within the Mexican-American community. This may have been the result of several interacting factors such as greater mobility of population, increased acculturation, presence of supermarkets, more youth-oriented clubs (YMCA, etc.), and recreational facilities/activities. Several respondents, however, made reference to this support system as playing a prominent role in meeting community instrumental and expressive needs. In short, the above elements of Hispanic NSS, with the exception of community leaders, fit well with the typology developed by Delgado and Humm-Delgado (1982).

How do Hispanic NSS function? This question attempts to identify the essential ingredients that make Hispanic natural support systems desirable and accessible to the Hispanic community. Culturally, Hispanics display a tendency to relate to individuals rather than institutions. When Hispanics seek assistance from formal institutions, it is the provider that they relate to and not the institution. Thus, when a highly regarded provider leaves an organization there is no guarantee that the person replacing him or her will pick up where he or she left off; this makes continuity-of-service provision difficult, if not impossible. Natural support providers have an ability to convey trust, respect, and loyalty, along with a willingness to accept consumers without morally prejudging them. This ability combined with a keen understanding of what is expected of them as providers, and accessibility (geographical, psychological, and logistical), allows natural support providers to exercise great influence in the help-seeking process.

How can Hispanic NSS be used in prevention? Hispanic NSS can provide a wide range of services that, when coordinated with substance abuse prevention efforts, can facilitate outreach into the community. NSS can provide transportation, information on community needs, referral, and space to hold groups/meetings, to list a few services. Prevention programs can also benefit from the "legitimacy" provided by influential community members. Prevention strategies can also assist in the formation of influential social support systems by linking families together who share similar needs

and concerns (mutual support type of groups). By having prevention programs actively utilizing Hispanic NSS, communities are
provided with an opportunity to control how services get conceptualized and implemented. In addition, it further highlights resources
that are present in the community—an important form of community empowerment.

Who can benefit? There is no target group (youth, parents, community) that cannot benefit from an active and formalized relationship between prevention programs and NSS. Youth benefit when
they are helped to feel that they belong to a community that still cares
about them. Parents, in turn, benefit when they are helped to feel less
isolated and given support and a sense of hope for the future. Communities benefit from having resources coordinated, thus reducing
waste and having services based upon their definition of need.

Training: Provision of training offers great potential in bringing
together formal providers and natural support providers. Training to
enhance awareness and skills related to the helping process can
foster collaboration. Training, however, must be thought of as addressing both NSS and formal systems. In short, it represents an
equal partnership. Staff must think not only of how to improve the
knowledge and skills of natural support providers; they, too, can
benefit from the wisdom of natural support providers. Training of
natural support providers, in turn, can have an important ripple
effect throughout the community.

Difficult to engage groups: Close collaboration between formal
systems and NSS, however, may not be possible with all groups and
situations. The identification and engagement of Hispanic NSS is
complex, labor-intensive, and very often requires excellent prob-
lem-solving skills on the part of staff, since this material is rarely
covered in formal education and workshops. Certain conditions do
not lend themselves to collaboration. Individuals/families heavily
involved in deviant behavior, or with strong negative peer networks, will prove difficult, or impossible, to assist with natural
supports. Youth who have lost trust in adults also represent a challenge, being beyond primary or secondary intervention, and in need
of treatment. One respondent noted that youth, in general, would
have little faith in natural supports as a result of being highly acculturated. Two respondents specifically noted that anyone can benefit,

regardless of age. Respondents went on to note that problems such as excessive use of alcohol by parents, child abuse, lack of financial resources, isolation, dysfunctional support groups such as gangs, and multiplicity of problems, hinder collaboration between Hispanic NSS and agencies.

Contextual considerations: Hispanic NSS are dynamic and ever-changing, impacted by population trends, density, and changing roles within the family. Consequently, it is important to take this into account in planning and intervention activities involving NSS. Rural/urban environments impact on how communities form and interact. Highly densely-populated communities, with rapidly shifting population groups, can result in feelings of anomie and disengagement among residents. Neighbors, for example, may only share geographical residence and little else, even if they belong to the same Hispanic subgroup. It is not uncommon to live in an area and not know one's neighbors. Situations like this do not lend themselves to active, caring social networks. Economic demands, in turn, may necessitate both parents working outside of the home. This phenomenon can also apply to godmothers, grandparents, and other significant family members, severely limiting their accessibility and ability to provide for expressive and instrumental needs.

Clearly, families are a central factor in Hispanic NSS. However, the community needs an extensive network of stable, intact families in order to sustain an active support system. Females play very important nurturance and helping roles within the family, perhaps as a result of tradition. Thus, a community experiencing rapid and dramatic disintegration will have a profound impact upon NSS; this situation is further compounded if females are bearing the brunt of the upheaval.

The process of acculturation will have an impact on the utilization of Hispanic NSS and needs to be taken into account in any form of assessment. Folk healers, for example, may prove to be an excellent resource for adults or elders, but not youth; the latter may find folk healers "foolish" and not to be taken seriously. Acculturation, as a result, may make it very difficult to engage youth when they consider most forms of NSS as outdated and from the "old country."

Organizational considerations: In turning to organizational factors that can severely limit collaboration with Hispanic NSS, two key areas emerge: (1) data gathering for the planning of collaborative activities; and (2) the importance of staff awareness, sensitivity, and skill in engaging and working with Hispanic NSS. Organizations need to develop methods for measuring utilization and existence/location of NSS. This will provide important data on service needs, gaps, identity of key natural support providers, and trends. However, for this to be accomplished, it will require major changes in intake forms, record keeping, and extensive documentation of the process used to involve NSS.

Staffing considerations: The hiring of Hispanic staff who are receptive to this intervention approach is crucial if collaboration is to succeed. Hispanic staff, and bilingual staff when it is not possible to hire the former, must have confidence in natural support providers, along with a willingness to accept these providers as peers. In addition, staff must be prepared to engage in a high degree of self-disclosure and be tested by natural support providers and the community. Bilingual, but not bicultural staff, may experience greater difficulty in working with NSS. They may have a command of the language but not the culture. Bilingual staff may have minimal or no awareness of Hispanic NSS, their function, and methods for engaging their support.

HOW HISPANIC NSS DIFFER FROM MORE CONVENTIONAL TYPES AND ANY SUBGROUP DIFFERENCES

In examining how Hispanic NSS differ from those of other groups, several unique characteristics of this group stand out. The definition of natural support systems provided by Baker (1977) is an excellent starting point for examining these differences, (1) personality of the natural support provider, (2) extended family, (3) self-definition and identity, (4) gender considerations, and (5) presence of community leaders.

1. *Personality of the natural support provider:* As already noted, the presence of Hispanic natural support systems such as religion, folk healing, etc., does not assure utilization. However, the individuals providing support must be competent, trustworthy, and accessible for the support system to be utilized. Hispanics, as noted, do not

necessarily relate to institutions, but to individuals employed within those settings. Consequently, the success or failure of a service/program is greatly contingent upon staffing.

2. *Extended family:* Baker's definition touches upon the importance of family. However, his definition does not make reference to extended family or families with open systems that allow nonblood relatives, etc., to become a prominent part of a family's constellation. The importance of the Hispanic family cannot be overly stressed. The review of the literature, responses from the questionnaire, and experiences related by field staff all indicate that Hispanic families must play a central role in any effort to involve the community. However, field staff must be flexible and have consumers define what family means to them rather than develop an institutional definition that may not be relevant to the Hispanic community they are attempting to reach.

3. *Self-definition and identity:* This dimension represents a dramatic departure from Baker's definition. Namely, that Hispanic NSS play an instrumental role in helping Hispanics maintain their identity through pride, development of a sense of control over their environment/needs, and providing role models for the community. These components form the cornerstone of any effort at developing empowerment in the community. In sum, Hispanic NSS provide for instrumental, expressive, and identity needs.

4. *Gender considerations:* The literature on Hispanics and human services is replete with examples indicating the importance of considering gender in the planning and delivery of services. Baker's definition does not note this factor, yet the literature and responses obtained in this study indicate that gender must be considered. The possibility of an appearance of impropriety, for example, a male natural support system provider helping a female, etc., could result in a barrier to the help-seeking process. Naturally, there are situations where this would not be an issue, i.e., male religious leader helping a female parishioner, etc.

5. *Presence of community leaders:* Hispanic community leaders are not necessarily a part of the natural support system, as it has been conceptualized in this report. Nevertheless, they represent an added dimension. They can be part of fulfilling a natural support-system-provider role like religious leader, merchant, etc., and in

addition, play a leadership role within the community that far exceeds their role as natural provider. Conversely, leaders, with their talents and altruism, can provide a voice for the community, but be natural support providers in the conventional sense. In essence, leadership may or may not be associated with traditional natural support provider roles and program staff must be able to differentiate between the two types.

In turning to Hispanic subgroup differences, the professional literature on Hispanics and human services highlights the importance of not "lumping" all Hispanic subgroups together, and the necessity to take into account the unique contribution each group makes. Consequently, this research project attempted to elicit responses as they applied to Mexicans, Puerto Ricans, and Cubans.

Remarkably, the mailed questionnaire did not uncover major differences among Hispanic subgroups, as was expected. In similar fashion to comments made in other sections of the questionnaire, respondents raised the importance of the family—many times from their own Hispanic subgroup perspectives. However, upon analysis, the factors/themes raised applied to all Hispanic groups. One difference, however, focused on types of folk healers listed, with each group having their "own," and various types of merchant organizations. The Cuban community has establishments that serve coffee; Mexican-American communities have places where "tacos" are sold; Puerto Rican communities have very specific types of grocery stores. Consequently, the question raised in this section of the questionnaire provided more in the area of similarities than differences.

CONCLUSION

There is little doubt that culture-specific service intervention with Hispanics is necessary. Further, it is widely acknowledged that the planning and delivery of said services is not easy, requiring a keen understanding of the community, and committed and competent staff to implement plans. The use of natural support systems represents one approach to bring close collaboration between community and agencies. This chapter has outlined a rationale for this approach and provided the reader with a variety of factors that must be taken into consideration.

References

Introduction

Frisbie, W.P. and Bean, F.D. (1995). The Latino family in comparative perspective: Trends and current conditions. In C.K. Jacobson (Ed.), *American families: Issues in race and ethnicity* (pp. 29-71). New York: Garland Publishing Inc.

Hurtado, A. (1995). Variations, combinations, and evolutions: Latino families in the United States. In R.E. Zambrana (Ed.), *Understanding Latino families: Scholarship, policy, and practice* (pp. 40-61). Thousand Oaks, CA: Sage Publications.

IPR Datanote. (1995). Puerto Ricans and other Latinos in the United States: March 1994. *Institute for Puerto Rican Policy*, 17, 1-2.

Ortiz, V. (1995). The study of Latino families: A point of departure. In R.E. Zambrana (Ed.), *Understanding Latino families: Scholarship, policy, and practice* (pp. 18-39). Thousand Oaks, CA: Sage Publications.

Pear, R. (December 4, 1992). New look at the U.S. in 2050: Bigger, older, and less white. *The New York Times*, A1, D18.

The New York Times. (April 22, 1994). Americans in 2020: Less white, more southern, 34.

Chapter 1

Albee, G.W. (1991). Reflections on macro-level prevention (interview). In J. Pransky (Ed.), *Prevention* (pp. 87-94). Springfield, MO: Paradigm Press.

Allen, R.L., and Allen, J.A. (1987). Sense of community, a shared vision and a positive culture: Core enabling factors in successful culture-based health promotion, *American Journal of Health Promotion*, Winter, 1-10.

Becerra, R.M., and Zambrana, R.M. (1985). Methodological approaches to research on Hispanics. *Social Work*, 30(1), 42-49.

Bell, R.A., Sunel, M., Aponte, J.F., Murrell, S.A., and Lin, E. (Eds.) (1983). *Assessing health and human service needs.* New York: Human Sciences Press.

Bernard, B. (1990). An overview of community-based prevention. In K.H. Rey, C.L. Faegre, and P. Lowery (Eds.), *Prevention Research Findings: 1988. OSAP Prevention Monograph-3* (pp. 126-147). Rockville, MD: OSAP.

Bloom, D., and Padilla, A.M. (1979). A peer interviewer model in conducting surveys among Mexican-American youth. *Journal of Community Psychology*, 7(2), 129-136.

Caplan, G., and Killilea, M. (Eds.) (1976). *Support systems and mutual help: Multidisciplinary explorations.* New York: Grune and Stratton.

Clayton, R.R. (1992). Transitions in drug use: Risk and protective factors. In M. Glantz and R. Pickens (Eds.), *Vulnerability to Drug Abuse* (pp. 15-52). Washington, DC: American Psychological Association.

Davis, L.V. (Ed.) (1994). *Building on women's strengths.* New York: The Haworth Press, Inc.

Delgado, M. (1979). A grass-roots model for needs assessment in Hispanic communities. *Child Welfare, 58*(9), 571-576.

Delgado, M. (1981). Using Hispanic adolescents to assess community needs. *Social Casework: The Journal of Contemporary Social Work, 62*(10), 607-613.

Delgado, M. (1994). Hispanic natural support systems and the AODA field: A developmental framework for collaboration. *Journal of Multicultural Social Work, 3*(2), 11-37.

Delgado, M. (1995a). Hispanic natural support systems and AOD services: Challenges and rewards for practice. *Alcoholism Treatment Quarterly, 12*(1), 17-31.

Delgado, M. (1995b). Natural support systems and AOD services to communities of color: A California case example. *Alcoholism Treatment Quarterly, 13*(4).

Delgado, M., and Humm-Delgado, D. (1982). Natural support systems: A source of strength in Hispanic communities. *Social Work, 27*(1), 83-90.

Delgado, M., and Humm-Delgado, D. (1993). Chemical dependence, self-help groups, and the Hispanic community. In R.S. Mayers, B.L. Kail, and T.D. Watts (Eds.), *Hispanic Substance Abuse* (pp. 145-146). Springfield, IL: Charles C Thomas Publishers.

Delgado, M., and Rosati, M. (1995). Religion, asset assessment and AOD: A case study of a Puerto Rican community in Massachusetts. *Journal of Health and Social Policy* (pending publication).

Dryfoos, J.G. (1990). *Adolescents at risk.* New York: Oxford University Press.

Eckenrode, J. (Ed.) (1991). *The social context of coping.* New York: Plenum Press.

Folkman, S., Chesney, M., McKusick, L.M., Ironson, G., Johnson, D.L., and Coates, T.J. (1991). Translating coping theory into an intervention. In J. Eckenrode (Ed.), *The social context of coping* (pp. 240-260). New York: Plenum Press.

Freeman, E.M. (1990). Social competence as a framework for addressing ethnicity and teenage alcohol problems. In A.R. Stiffman and L.E. Davis (Eds.), *Ethnic issues in adolescent mental health* (pp. 247-266). Newbury Park, CA: Sage Publications.

Gfroerer, J., and De La Rosa, M. (1993). Protective and risk factors associated with drug use among Hispanic youth. *Journal of Addictive Diseases, 12*(2), 87-107.

Gutierrez, L.M. (1992). Empowering ethnic minorities in the twenty-first century: The role of human service organizations. In Y. Hasenfield (Ed.), *Human services as complex organizations* (pp. 320-338). Newbury Park, CA: Sage Publications.

Hawkins, J.D., Lishner, D.M., and Catalano, F. Jr. (1985). Childhood predictors and the prevention of adolescent substance abuse. In C.L. Jones and R.J. Battles (Eds.), *Etiology of drug abuse: Implications for prevention* (pp. 75-126). National Institute on Drug Abuse Research Monograph 56. DHHS Pub. No. (ADM) 87-1335. Washington, DC: U.S. Government Printing Office.

Holmes, G.E. (1992). Social work research and the empowerment paradigm. In D.S. Saleebey (Ed.), *The strengths perspective in social work practice* (pp. 158-168). New York: Longman Publishers.

Humm-Delgado, D., and Delgado, M. (1983). Assessing Hispanic mental health needs: Issues and recommendations. *Journal of Community Psychology, 11*(4), 363-375.

Humm-Delgado, D., and Delgado, M. (1986). Gaining community entree to assess service needs of Hispanics. *Social Casework: The Journal of Contemporary Social Work, 67*(2), 80-89.

Hutcheson, J.S., and Prather, J.E. (1988). Community mobilization and participation in the zoning process. *Urban Affairs Quarterly, 23*(3), 346-368.

Krimsky, S., and Golding, D. (Eds.) (1992). *Social theories of risk.* Westport, CT: Praeger Press.

Kumpfer, K.L. (1987). Special populations: Etiology and prevention of vulnerability to chemical dependency in children of substance abusers. In B.S. Brown and A.R. Mills (Eds.), *Youth at risk for substance abuse* (pp. 1-72). National Institute on Drug Abuse. DHHS Pub. No. (ADM) 90-1537. Washington, DC: U.S. Government Printing Office.

Marin, G. (1993). Defining culturally appropriate interventions: Hispanics as a case study. *Journal of Community Psychology, 21*(2), 149-161.

Marin, G., and Marin, B.V. (1991). *Research with Hispanic populations.* Newbury Park, CA: Sage Publications.

Marti-Costa, S., and Serrano-Garcia, I. (1987). Needs assessment and community development: An ideological perspective. In F.M. Cox, J.L. Erlich, J. Rothman, and J.E. Tropman (Eds.), *Strategies of community organization* (pp. 362-373). Itasca, IL: F.E. Peacock Publishers, Inc.

The Maurico Gaston Institute of Latino Community Development and Public Policy. (1992). *Latinos in Holyoke, Massachusetts.* Boston: University of Massachusetts.

McKnight, J.L., and Kretzmann, J. (1991). *Mapping Community Capacity.* Evanston, IL: Center for Urban Affairs Policy and Research, Northwestern University.

McPhillip, J. (1987). *Need analysis: Tools for the human services and education.* Newbury Park, CA: Sage Publications.

McWhirter, J.J., McWhirter, B.T., McWhirter, A.M., and McWhirter, E.H. (1993). *At-risk youth: A comprehensive response.* Pacific Grove, CA: Brooks/Cole.

Nadel, A., and Morales-Nadel, M. (1993). Multiculturalism in urban schools: A Puerto Rican perspective. In S.W. Rothstein (Ed.), *Handbook of schooling in urban America* (pp. 145-159). Westport, CT: Greenwood Press.

Newcomb, M.D. (1992). Understanding the multi-dimensional nature of drug use and abuse: The role of consumption, risk factors, and protective factors. In M.

Glantz and R. Pickens (Eds.), *Vulnerability to drug use* (pp. 255-298), Washington, DC: American Psychological Association.

Nisbet, J. (Ed.) (1992). *Natural supports in school, at work, and in the community for people with disabilities.* Baltimore, MD: Paul Brooks Publisher.

Padilla, E.R., Padilla, A.M., Ramirez, R., Morales, A., and Olmeda, E.L. (1979). Inhalant, marijuana, and alcohol abuse among barrio children and adolescents. *International Journal of the Addictions, 17*(7), 945-964.

Perez, R., Padilla, A.M., Ramirez, A., Ramirez, R., and Rodriguez, M. (1980). Correlates and changes over time in drug and alcohol abuse within a barrio population. *American Journal of Community Psychology, 8*(6), 621-636.

Rhodes, J.E., and Jason, L.A. (1988). *Preventing substance abuse among children and adolescents.* New York: Pergamon Press.

Rutter, M. (1987). Psychological resilience and protective mechanisms. *American Journal of Orthopsychiatry, 37*, 317-331.

Saleebey, D.S. (Ed.) (1992). *The strengths perspective in social work practice.* New York: Longman Publishers.

Streeter, C.L., and Franklin, C. (1992). Defining and measuring social support: Guidelines for social work practitioners. *Research on Social Work Practice, 2*(1), 81-98.

Sullivan, W.P. (1992). Reconsidering the environment as a helping resource. In D.S. Saleebey (Ed.), *The strengths perspective in social work practice* (pp. 148-157). New York: Longman.

Weber, G.H. (1982). Self-help and beliefs. In G.H. Weber, and L.M. Cohen (Eds.), *Beliefs and self-help* (pp. 13-30). New York: Human Sciences Press.

Werner, G.H. (1991). *Against the odds.* Ithaca, NY: Cornell University Press.

Chapter 2

Ball, M.B. and Whittington, F.J. (1995). *Surviving dependence: Voices of African-American elders.* Amityville, NY: Baywood Publishing Co., Inc.

Barresi, C.M. and Skinner, J.H. (1994). Overview of health and minority elders: Implications for practice, management, policy, and research. In. C.M. Barresi (Ed.), *Health and minority elders: An analysis of applied literature, 1980-1990* (pp. 3-21). Washington, DC: American Association of Retired Persons.

Barresi, C.M. and Stull, D.E. (1993). *Ethnic elderly and long-term care.* New York: Springer Publishing Co.

Bartlett, M. and Font, M.E. (1995). Hispanic men and long-term care: The wives' perspective. *Journal of Multicultural Social Work, 3*, 77-88.

Bastida, E. and Lueders, L. (1994). Hispanic elderly health: An overview of the literature. In C.M. Barresi (Ed.), *Health and minority elders: An analysis of applied literature, 1980-1990* (pp.77-97). Washington, DC: American Association of Retired Persons.

Becerra, R.M. and Zambrana, R.E. (1985). Methodological approaches to research on Hispanics. *Social Work, 30*, 42-49.

Capitman, J.A., Hernandez-Gallegos, W., and Yee, D.L. (1992). Diversity assessments in aging services. In E.P. Stanford and F. Torres-Gil (Eds.), *Diversity: New approaches to ethnic minority aging* (pp.143-154). Amityville, NY: Baywood Publishing Co., Inc.

Chavis, D.M. and Wandersman, A. (1990). Sense of community in the urban environment: A catalyst for participation and community development. *American Journal of Community Psychology, 18*, 55-80.

Coke, M.M. and Twaite, J.A. (1995). *The Black elderly: Satisfaction and quality of later life.* Binghamton, NY: The Haworth Press, Inc.

Dean, D.L. (1994). How to use focus groups. In J.S. Wholey, H.P. Hatry, and K.E. Newcomer (Eds.), *Handbook of practical program evaluation* (pp. 338-349). San Francisco, CA: Jossey-Bass Publishers.

Delgado, M. (1995). Puerto Rican elders and natural support systems: Implications for human services. *Journal of Gerontological Social Work, 24*, 115-130.

Delgado, M. (In press, a). Aging research and the Puerto Rican community: The use of an advisory committee of intended respondents. *The Gerontologist.*

Delgado, M. (In press, b). Puerto Rican elders and botanical shops: A community resource or liability? *Social Work in Health Care.*

Delgado, M. (In press, c). Puerto Rican food establishments as social service organizations: Results of an asset assessment. *Journal of Community Practice.*

Delgado, M. (In press, d). Puerto Rican elders and merchant establishments: Natural caregiving systems or simply businesses? *Journal of Health and Social Policy.*

Delgado, M. (under review, a). Interpretation of Puerto Rican elder research findings: A community forum of research respondents.

Delgado, M. (under review, b). Religion as a caregiving system for Puerto Rican elders with functional disabilities.

Delgado, M. and Tennstedt, S. (under review). Making the case for culturally appropriate community services: Puerto Rican elders and their caregivers.

Espino, D.V. (1993). Hispanic elderly and long-term care: Implications for ethnically sensitive services. In C.M. Barresi and D.E. Stull (Eds.), *Ethnic elderly and long-term care.* New York: Springer Publishing Co.

Garcia, J.L. (1985). A needs assessment of elderly Hispanics in an inner-city senior citizen complex: Implications for practice. *Journal of Applied Gerontology, 4*, 72-85.

Gaston Institute. (1992). *Latinos in Springfield.* Boston, MA: University of Massachusetts.

Gaston Institute. (1994). *Latinos in Springfield: Poverty, income, education, employment, and housing.* Boston, MA: University of Massachusetts.

Hayes-Bautista, D.E. (1992). Young Latinos, older Anglos, and public policy: Lessons from California. In E.P. Stanford and F. Torres-Gil (Eds.), *Diversity: New approaches to ethnic minority aging* (pp.73-80). Amityville, NY: Baywood Publishing Co., Inc.

Heath, S.B. and McLaughlin, M.W. (1993). *Identity and inner-city youth: Beyond ethnicity and gender.* New York: Teachers College Press.

Henderson, J.N. (1994). Ethnic and racial issues. In J.F. Gubrium and A. Sankar (Eds.), *Qualitative methods in aging research* (pp. 33-50). Thousand Oaks, CA: Sage Publications.

Holmes, E.R. and Holmes, L.D. (1995). *Other cultures, elder years.* Thousand Oaks, CA: Sage Publications.

Jimenez, R.G. and de Figueiredo, J.M. (1994). Issues in the psychiatric care of Hispanic American elders. In *Ethnic minority elderly: A task force report of the American Psychiatric Association* (pp. 63-89). Washington, DC: American Psychiatric Association.

Krueger, R.A. (1988). *Focus groups: A practical guide for applied research.* Newbury Park, CA: Sage Publications.

Lee, J.A.B. (1994). *The empowerment approach to social work practice.* New York: Columbia University.

Marin, G. and Marin, B.O. (1991). *Research with Hispanic populations.* Newbury Park, CA: Sage Publications.

Marti-Costa, S. and Serrano-Garcia, I. (1995). Needs assessment and community development: An ideological perspective. In. F.M. Cox, J.L. Erlich, J. Rothman, and J.E. Tropman (Eds.), *Strategies of community organization* (pp. 257-267). Itasca, IL: F.E. Peacock Publishers, Inc.

McKillip, J. (1987). *Needs analysis: Tools for the human services and education.* Newbury Park, CA: Sage Publications.

McKnight, J.L. and Kretzmann, J.P. (1990). *Mapping community capacity.* Evenston, IL: Center for Urban Affairs and Policy Research, Northwestern University.

Ragin, C.C. and Hein, J. (1993). The comparative study of ethnicity: Methodological and conceptual issues. In J.H. Stanfield II and R.M. Dennis (Eds.), *Race and ethnicity in research methods* (pp. 254-272). Thousand Oaks, CA: Sage Publications.

Roberts, S. (Sunday, October 9, 1994). Hispanic population outnumbers blacks in four cities as nation's demographics shift. *The New York Times,* 34.

Sánchez, C. (1987). Self-help: Model for strengthening the informal support system of the Hispanic elderly. *Journal of Gerontological Social Work,* 9, 117-130.

Sánchez-Ayéndez, M. (1988). Puerto Rican elderly women: The cultural dimension of social support network. *Women and Health,* 14, 239-252.

Soriano, F.I. (1995). *Conducting needs assessments: A multidisciplinary approach.* Thousand Oaks, CA: Sage Publications.

Sotomayor, M. and Curiel, H. (Eds.). (1988). *Hispanic elderly: A cultural signature.* Edinburg, TX: Pan American University Press.

Stanford, E. P. and Torres-Gil, F. (Eds.). (1992). *Diversity: New approaches to ethnic minority aging.* Amityville, NY: Baywood Publishing Co., Inc.

Treas, J. (1995). Older Americans in the 1990s and beyond. *Population Bulletin,* 50, 2.

Witkin, B.R. and Altschuld, J.W. (1995). *Planning and conducting needs assessments: A practical guide.* Thousand Oaks, CA: Sage Publication.

Chapter 3

Bartlett, M.C. and Font, M.E. (1994). Hispanic men and long-term care: The wives' perspective. *Journal of Multicultural Social Work*, 3, 77-88.

Bastida, E. (1988). Reexamining assumptions about extended familism: Older Puerto Ricans in a comparative perspective. In M. Sotomayor and H. Curiel (Eds.), *Hispanic elderly: A cultural signature* (pp. 163-183). Edinburg, TX: Pan American University Press.

Bastida, E. and Lueders, L. (1994). Hispanic elderly health: An overview of the literature. In C.M. Barresi (Ed.), *Health and minority elders: An analysis of applied literature, 1980-1990* (pp. 77-97). Washington, DC: American Association of Retired Persons.

Becerra, R.M. and Shaw, D. (1984). *The Hispanic elderly: A research reference guide*. New York: University Press of America.

Blackwell, J.E. (1985). *The Black community*. New York: Harper and Row.

Caraballo, E.R. (1990). *The role of the Pentecostal church as a service provider in the Puerto Rican community of Boston, Massachusetts: A case study*. Waltham, MA: Brandeis University.

Chatters, L. and Taylor, R. (1989). Age differences in religious participation among Black adults. *Journals of Gerontology: Social Sciences*, 44, S183-189.

Coke, M.M. and Twaite, J.A. (1995). *The Black elderly: Satisfaction and quality of later life*. Binghamton, NY: The Haworth Press, Inc.

Cox, H. (1995). *Fire from heaven: The rise of Pentecostal spirituality and the reshaping of religion in the twenty-first century*. Reading, MA: Addison-Wesley Publishing Co.

Cruz-Lopez, M. and Pearson, R.E. (1985). The support needs and resources of Puerto Rican elders. *The Gerontologist*, 25, 483-487.

Delgado, M. (1997). Interpretation of Puerto Rican elder research findings: A community forum of research respondents. *The Journal of Applied Gerontology*, 16, 317-332.

Delgado, M. (1996). Puerto Rican elders and botanical shops: A community resource or liability? *Social Work in Health Care*, 23(1), 67-81.

Delgado, M. (1995). Puerto Rican elders and natural support systems. *Journal of Gerontological Social Work*, 24, 115-130.

Delgado, M. (1982). Hispanic elderly and natural support systems: A special focus on Puerto Ricans. *Journal of Geriatric Psychiatry*, 15, 239-251.

Delgado, M. and Rosati, M. (pending publication). Religion, asset assessment and AOD: A case study of a Puerto Rican community in Massachusetts. *Journal of Health and Social Policy*.

Delgado, M. and Tennstedt, S. (pending publication). Puerto Rican elder caregivers in a New England community. *Health and Social Work*.

Gaiter, D.J. (December 24, 1980). At Christmas, Hispanic Pentecostal church puts stress on "gifts" without price tags. *The New York Times*, B1, B4.

Gallego, D.T. (1988). Religiosity as a coping mechanism among Hispanic elderly. In M. Sotomayor and H. Curiel (Eds.), *Hispanic elderly: A cultural signature* (pp. 117-135). Edinburg, TX: Pan American University Press.

Gelfand, D.E. (1994). *Aging and ethnicity.* New York: Springer Publishing Co.

Hamilton, C.V. (1972). *The Black preacher in America.* New York: William Morrow and Co., Inc.

Holmes, E.R. and Holmes, L.D. (1995). *Other cultures, elder years.* Thousand Oaks, CA: Sage Publications.

Lindholm, K.J., Marin, G., and Lopez, R.E. (1980). *Fundamentals of proposal writing: A guide for minority researchers.* Rockville, MD: National Institute of Mental Health.

Niebuhr, G. (December 11, 1994). A ceremony in Mexico City shows growth in mormonism. *The New York Times*, 36.

Saleebey, D.S. (Ed.). (1992). *The strengths perspective in social work practice.* New York: Longman Publishers.

Sánchez, C. (1990). Sistemas de apoyo informal de viudas mayores de 60 anos en Puerto Rico. *Revista Salud y Cultura*, 12, 101-115.

Sánchez, C. (1987). Self-help: Model for strengthening the informal support system of the Hispanic elderly. *Journal of Gerontological Social Work*, 9, 117-130.

Sánchez-Ayéndez, M. (1988). Puerto Rican elderly women: The cultural dimension of social support network. *Women and Health*, 14, 239-252.

Stevens-Arroyo, A.M. and Stevens-Diaz, A.M. (1993). Latino churches and schools as urban battlefields. In S.W. Rothstein (Ed.), *Handbook of schooling in urban America* (pp. 245-270). Westport, CT: Greenwood Press.

Tye, L. (November 13, 1994a). Faith, hope and multitudes: Across nations, races, Pentecostal gains 50,000 members per day. *The Boston Globe*, 1, 28, 29.

Tye, L. (November 14, 1994b). Pentecostal world reach: Faith finds millions underground in China. *The Boston Globe*, 1, 7, 8.

Tye, L. (November 15, 1994c). Brazil's poor hear Pentecostalism's call. *The Boston Globe*, 1, 16, 17.

Tye, L. (November 16, 1994d). Pentecostalism's U.S. crossroads. *The Boston Globe*, 1, 20, 21.

Chapter 4

Agins, T. (March 15, 1985). To Hispanics in U.S., a bodega, or grocery, is a vital part of life. *The Wall Street Journal,* 1, 6, 13.

Aldrich, H. E. and Waldinger, R. (1990). Ethnicity and entrepreneurship. *Annual Review of Sociology,* 16, 111-135.

Allen, R. L. and Allen, J. A. (1987). A sense of community, a shared vision, and a positive culture: Core enabling factors in successful culture based health promotion. *American Journal of Health Promotion, Winter,* 1-10.

Burros, M. (July 18, 1990). Supermarkets reach out to Hispanic customers. *The New York Times,* C1, C6.

Carmody, D. (May 2, 1972). Bodega owners gain strength in co-op here. *The New York Times,* 31.

Castex, G. M. (1994). Providing services to Hispanic/Latino populations. *Social Work,* 39, 288-296.

Collins, A. H. and Pancoast, D. L. (1976). *Natural helping networks: A strategy for prevention.* Washington, DC: National Association of Social Workers.

Cross, T. L. (1988). Services to minority populations: Cultural competence continuum. *Focal Point,* 3, 1-4.

Daley, J. M. and Wong, P. (1994). Community development with emerging ethnic communities. *Journal of Community Practice,* 1, 9-24.

De La Rosa, M. (1988). Natural support systems of Hispanic Americans: A key dimension of well-being. *Health and Social Work,* 13, 181-190.

Delgado, M. (pending publication, a). Puerto Rican elders and natural support systems: Implications for human services. *Journal of Gerontological Social Work.*

Delgado, M. (pending publication, b). Community asset assessment and substance abuse prevention: A case study involving the Puerto Rican community. *Journal of Child and Adolescent Substance Abuse.*

Delgado, M. (pending review). Puerto Rican elders and merchant establishments: Natural support systems or simply businesses?

Delgado, M. (1994). Hispanic natural support systems and the alcohol and drug abuse field: A developmental framework for collaboration. *Journal of Multicultural Social Work.*

Delgado, M. (1982). Hispanic elderly and natural support systems: A special focus on Puerto Ricans. *Journal of Geriatric Psychiatry,* 15, 239-251.

Delgado, M. and Humm-Delgado, D. (1982). Natural support systems: Source of strength in Hispanic communities. *Social Work,* 27, 83-89.

Delgado, M. and Rosati, M. (pending review). Religion, asset assessment and AOD: A case study of a Puerto Rican community in Massachusetts.

Evans, S. M. and Boyte, H. C. (1986) *Free spaces: The sources of change in America.* New York: Harper and Row.

Fisher, R. and Kling, J. M. (1987). Leading people: Two approaches to the role of ideology in community organizing. *Radical America,* 21, 31-45.

Fitzpatrick, J. P. (1987). *Puerto Rican Americans: The meaning of migration to the mainland.* Englewood Cliffs, NJ: Prentice-Hall.

Florin, P. and Wandersman, A. (1990). An introduction to citizen participation, voluntary organizations, and community development: Insights for empowerment through research. *American Journal of Community Psychology,* 18, 41-53.

Gaston Institute. (1992). *Latinos in Holyoke.* Boston, MA: University of Massachusetts.

Gaston Institute. (1994). *Latinos in Holyoke: Poverty, income, education, employment, and housing.* Boston, MA: University of Massachusetts.

Glugoski, G., Reisch, M., and Rivera, F. G. (1994). A wholistic ethno-cultural paradigm: A new model for community organization teaching and practice. *Journal of Community Practice,* 1, 81-98.

Gonzalez, D. (September 1, 1992). Dominican immigration alters Hispanic New York. *The New York Times,* Section A, 1.

Gottlieb, B. H. (Ed.) (1981). *Social networks and social support.* Beverly Hills, CA: Sage Publications.

Gottlieb, B. H. (1988). *Marshaling social support: Formats, processes and effects.* Newbury Park, CA: Sage Publications.

Gutierrez, L. M. and Ortega, R. M. (1991). Developing methods to empower Latinos: The importance of groups. *Social Work With Groups,* 14, 23-43.

Gutierrez, L., Ortega, R. M., and Suarez, Z. (1990). Self-help and the Latino community. In T. J. Powell (Ed.), *Working with self-help* (pp. 218-236). Silver Springs, MD: National Association of Social Workers.

Hernandez, R. (1994, July 12). Where Hispanic merchants thrive: In Westchester, growth of businesses bolsters economy. *The New York Times,* 1.

Howe, M. (1986, November 19). Bodegas find prosperity amid change. *The New York Times,* 8.

Korrol, V. E. S. (1983). *From colonia to community: The history of Puerto Ricans in New York City, 1917-1948.* Westport, CT: Greenwood Press.

Kretzmann, J. P. and McKnight, J. L. (1993). *Building communities from the inside out: A path toward finding and mobilizing a community's assets.* Evanston, IL: Center for Urban Affairs and Policy Research, Northwestern University.

Levine, R. (1990, July 30). The new arrivals; immigrants reshape New York: Young immigrant wave lifts New York economy. *The New York Times,* 1.

Mason, J. L. (1994). Developing culturally competent organizations. *Focal Point,* 8, 1-7.

McKnight, J. L. and Kretzmann, J. (1991) *Mapping community capacity.* Evanston, IL.: Center for Urban Affairs and Policy Research, Northwestern University.

McLaughlin, M. W., Irby, M. A., and Langman, J. (1994). *Urban sanctuaries: Neighborhood organizations in the lives and futures of inner-city youth.* San Francisco, CA; Jossey-Bass Publications.

Pearson, R. E. (1990). *Counseling and social support: Perspectives and practice.* Newbury Park, CA: Sage Publications.

Raynor, V. (1991, July 7). Charting the migration of Puerto Ricans, and their resilience. *The New York Times,* 14.

Rierden, A. (1992, February 16). Problems temper Puerto Rican's success. *The New York Times,* Section 12 CN, 1.

Rohter, L. (1985a, August 11). New York's thriving Hispanic banks. *The New York Times,* 4.

Rohter, L. (1985b, October 10). El Barrio residents worry and wait. *The New York Times,* Section B, 16.

Rutter, M. (1987). Psychological resilience and protective mechanisms. *American Journal of Orthopsychiatry,* 37, 317-331.

Sánchez, A. (1988). Puerto Rican elderly women: The cultural dimension of social support network. *Women and Health,* 14, 239-252.

Sánchez-Ayéndez, C. (1987). Self-help: Model for strengthening the informal support system of the Hispanic elderly. *Journal of Gerontological Social Work,* 9, 117-130.

Sarason, Y. and Koberg, C. (1994). Hispanic women small business owners. *Hispanic Journal of Behavioral Sciences,* 16, 355-360.

Stout, H. (June 26, 1988). What's new in Hispanic business: Out of the Barrio and into the mainstream. *The New York Times,* 13.

Suarez, Z. E. (1992). Use of self-care by Hispanics: Culture, access or need? *Journal of Health and Social Policy,* 4, 31-45.

Terry, S. (1992, August 22). A wave of immigration is fast changing Boston. *The New York Times,* 5.

U.S. Bureau of the Census (1991). *The Hispanic population in the United States: March 1990* (Current Population Reports, Series p-20, No. 449). Washington, DC: U.S. Government Printing Office.

Valle, R. and Vega, W. (Eds.) (1980). *Hispanic natural support systems.* Sacramento, CA: State of California.

Vazquez, J. D. (1974). La bodega—A social institution. *In the Puerto Rican curriculum development workshop: A report* (pp. 31-36). New York: *Council on Social Work Education.*

Whittaker, J. K. and Garbarino, J. (Eds.) (1983). *Social support networks: Informal helping in the human services.* New York: Aldine Publishing Co.

Chapter 5

Borrello, M.A. and Mathias, E. (1977). Botanicas: Puerto Rican folk pharmacies. *Natural History,* 86, 64-73.

Cruz-Lopez, M. and Pearson, R.E. (1985). The support needs and resources of Puerto Rican elderly. *The Gerontologist,* 25, 483-487.

Delgado, M. (pending publication a). Puerto Rican elders and natural support systems: Implications for human services. *Journal of Gerontological Social Work.*

Delgado, M. (pending publication b). Natural support systems and AOD services to communities of color: A California case example. *Alcoholism Treatment Quarterly.*

Delgado, M. (1995). Hispanic natural support systems and AOD services: Challenges and rewards for practice. *Alcoholism Treatment Quarterly,* 12, 17-31.

Delgado, M. (1994). Hispanic natural support systems and the alcohol and drug abuse field: A developmental framework for collaboration. *Journal of Multi-Cultural Social Work,* 3, 11-37.

Delgado, M. (1982). Hispanic elderly and natural support systems: A special focus on Puerto Ricans. *Journal of Geriatric Psychiatry,* 15, 239-251.

Delgado, M. (1979). Herbal medicine in the Puerto Rican community. *Health and Social Work,* 4, 24-40.

Delgado, M. and Humm-Delgado, D. (1982). Natural support systems: Source of strength in Hispanic communities. *Social Work,* 27, 83-89.

Espino, D.V. (1993). Hispanic elderly and long-term care: Implications for ethnically sensitive services. In C.M. Barresi and D.E. Stull (Eds.), *Ethnic elderly and long-term care* (pp. 101-112). New York: Springer Publishing Co.

Fetherston, D. (August 17, 1992). Shop where business is a religion. *Newsday,* 33.

Fisch, S. (1968). Botanicas and spiritism in a metropolis. Milbank Memorial Fund, 41, 377-388.

Gallagher, S.K. (1994). *Older people giving care.* Westport, CT: Auburn House.

Harwood, A. (1981). Mainland Puerto Ricans. In A. Harwood (Ed.), *Ethnicity and medical care* (pp. 397-481). Cambridge, MA: Harvard University Press.

Harwood, A. (1977). *Rx: Spiritist as needed: A study of a Puerto Rican community mental health resource.* New York: John Wiley and Sons.

Helfound, D. (July 28, 1994). Faith in folk remedies; many immigrants trust their well-being to spiritual healers. *The Los Angeles Times*, 6.

Mahard, R. (1989). Elderly Puerto Rican women in the continental United States. In C.T. Garcia and M.L. Mattei (Eds.), *The psychosocial development of Puerto Rican women* (pp. 243-260). New York: Praeger Press.

Montana, C. (August 25, 1991). Unconventional wisdom has it some Hispanics put faith in ancient, unusual rites. *Chicago Tribune*, 1.

Pachter, L.M. (1994). Culture and clinical care: Folk illness beliefs and behaviors and their implication for health care delivery. *Journal of American Medical Association*, vol. 271, no. 9, (pp. 690-694).

Sánchez, C. (1990). Sistemas de apoyo informal de viudas mayores de 60 años en Puerto Rico. *Revista Salud Y Cultura*, 10, 101-115.

Sánchez, C. (1987). Self-help: Model for strengthening the informal support system of the Hispanic elderly. *Journal of Gerontological Social Work*, 9, 117-130.

Sánchez-Ayéndez, M. (1992). Older and middle-aged Puerto Rican women: Cultural components of support networks. Paper presented at the American Anthropological Association Annual Meeting, San Francisco, CA.

Sánchez-Ayéndez, M. (1988). Puerto Rican elderly women: The cultural dimension of social support network. *Women and Health*, 14, 239-252.

Spencer-Molloy, F. (March 2, 1994). Doctor negotiates path between folk and traditional medicines. *The Hartford Courant*, D9.

Valdes, A. (December 15, 1994). A faith emerges from the shadows. *The Boston Globe*, 74, 78.

Chapter 6

De La Cancela, V. and Zavala-Martinez, I. An analysis of culturalism in Latino mental health: Folk medicine as a case in point. *Hispanic Journal of Behavioral Sciences* 5: 251-274.

Delgado, M. (forthcoming publication). Hispanic natural support systems and AODA services: Challenges and rewards for practice. *Alcoholism Treatment Quarterly.*

Delgado, M. (1979-1980). Accepting folk healers: Problems and rewards. *Journal of Social Welfare* 6: 5-16.

Delgado, M. (1982). Use of key informants in assessing Hispanic mental health needs. *Journal of Mental Health Administration* 9: 2-4.

Delgado, M. (1986) Puerto Ricans. *18th Edition of the Encyclopedia of Social Work.* New York: National Association of Social Workers.

Delgado, M. (1989) Alcoholism treatment and Hispanic youth, in R. Wright Jr. and T.D. Watts (Eds.). *Alcohol problems of minority youth in America.* Lewiston: The Edwin Mellon Press.

Delgado, M. and Humm-Delgado, D. (1980). Interagency collaboration to increase resources in serving Hispanics. *Hispanic Journal of Behavioral Sciences,* 2, 269-285.

Delgado, M. and Humm-Delgado, D. (1993). Chemical dependence, self-help groups, and the Hispanic community. In R.S. Mayers, B.L. Kail, and T.D. Watts (Eds.). *Hispanic substance abuse* (pp. 145-156), Springfield, IL: Charles C Thomas.

Delgado, M. and Humm-Delgado, D. (pending publication). Chemical dependence, self-help groups, and the Hispanic community. In R.S. Mayers, B.L. Kail, and T.D. Watts (Eds.). *Hispanic substance abuse.* Springfield, IL: Charles C Thomas.

Delgado, M. and Rodriguez-Andrew, S. (1991). *Alcohol and other drug use among Hispanic youth.* OSAP Technical Report 4. Rockville, MD: Office of Substance Abuse Prevention.

Fitzpatrick, J.P. (1990). Addiction prevention and correction among Puerto Ricans: The cultural and social context. In R. Glick and J. Moore (Eds.). *Drugs in Hispanic communities.* New Brunswick, ME: Rutgers University Press.

Froland, C., Pancoast, D.L., Chapman, N.J., and Kimboko, P.J. (1981). *Helping networks and human services.* Beverly Hills, CA: Sage Publications.

Gans, S. and Horton, G.T. (1975). *Integration of human services: The state and municipal levels.* New York: Praeger Publishers.

Glick, R. and Moore, J. *Drugs in Hispanic communities.* New Brunswick, ME: Rutgers University Press.

Humm-Delgado, D. and Delgado, M. (1983). Assessing Hispanic mental health needs: Issues and approaches. *Journal of Community Psychology* 11: 363-375.

Humm-Delgado, D. and Delgado, M. (1986). Gaining community entree to assess service needs of Hispanics. *Social Casework* 67: 80-89.

Kraus, W.A. (1984). *Collaboration in organizations: Alternatives to hierarchy.* New York: Human Sciences Press, Inc..

Lenrow, P.B. and Burch, R.W. (1981). Mutual aid and professional services: Opposing or complementary? In B.H. Gottlieb (Ed.). *Social networks and social support.* Beverly Hills, CA: Sage Publications.

Mayers, R.S., Kail, B.L., and Watts, T.D. (Eds.) (1992). *Hispanic substance abuse.* Springfield, IL: Charles C Thomas.

Rio, A., Santisteban, D.A., and Szapocznik, J. Treatment approaches for hispanic drug-abusing adolescents. In R. Glick and J. Moore (Eds.) *Drugs in Hispanic communities.* New Brunswick, ME: Rutgers University Press.

Singer, M. and Borrero, M. (1984). Indigenous treatment for alcoholism: The Case of Puerto Rican Spiritism. *Medical Anthropology* 8: 246-273.

Singer, M., Davison, L., and Yalin, F. (1987). *Conference proceedings: Alcohol use and abuse among Hispanic adolescents.* Hartford, CT: Hispanic Health Council.

Valle, R. (1980). A natural resource system for health-mental health promotion to Latino/Hispano populations. In R. Valle and W. Vega (Eds.). *Hispanic natural support systems: Mental health promotion strategies.* Sacramento, CT: State of California.

Velez, C.G. (1980). Mexicano/Hispano support systems and confianza: Theoretical issues of cultural adaptation. In R. Valle and W. Vega (Eds.) *Hispanic natural support systems: Mental health promotion strategies.* Sacramento, CA: State of California.

Weber, G.H. (1982). Self-help and beliefs. In G.H. Weber and L.M Cohen (Eds.) *Beliefs and self-help.* New York: Human Sciences Press.

Whittaker, J.K. (1983). Mutual helping in human service practice. In J.K. Whittaker and J. Garbarino (Eds.) *Social support networks: Informal helping in the human services.* New York: Aldine Publishing Co.

Chapter 7

Baker, F. (1977). The interface between professional and natural support systems. *Clinical Social Work Journal* 5: 139-148.

Bernal, G. and Flores-Ortiz, Y. (1982). Latino families in therapy: Engagement and evaluation. *Journal of Marital and Family Therapy* 8: 357-365.

De La Cancela, V. and Zavala-Martinez, I. (1983). An analysis of culturalism in Latino mental health: Folk medicine as a case in point. *Hispanic Journal of Behavioral Sciences* 5: 251-274.

De La Rosa, M. (1988). Natural support systems of Puerto Ricans: A key dimension of well being. *Health and Social Work* 13: 181-190.

Delgado, M. (1989). Alcoholism treatment and Hispanic youth. In R. Wright Jr. and T.D. Watts (Eds.). *Alcohol Problems of Minority Youth in America.* Lewiston, ME: The Edwin Mellon Press.

Delgado, M. (1995). Hispanics/Latinos. In J. Phillead and F.L. Brisbane (Eds.). *cultural competence for social workers: A guide for alcohol and other drug abuse prevention professionals working with ethnic/racial communities* (pp. 43-67). Rockville, MD: Center on Substance Abuse Prevention.

Delgado, M. and Humm-Delgado, D. (1980). Interagency collaboration to increase community resources in serving Hispanics. *Hispanic Journal of Behavioral Sciences,* 2: 269-286.

Delgado, M. and Humm-Delgado, D. (1982). Natural support systems: Source of strength in Hispanic communities. *Social Work* 27: 83-89.

Delgado, M. and Rodriguez-Andrew, S. (1991). *Alcohol and other drug use among Hispanic youth.* OSAP Technical Report 4. Rockville, MD: Office of Substance Abuse Prevention.

Froland, C., Pancoast, D.L., Chapman, N.J., and Kimboko, P.K. (1981). *Helping networks and human services.* Beverly Hills, CA: Sage Publications.

Garbarino, J. (1983). Social support networks: RX for the helping professionals. In J.K. Whittaker and J. Garbarino (Eds.). *Social support networks: Informal helping in the human services.* New York: Aldine Publishing Co.

Hayes-Bautista, D.E., Schink, W.O., and Chapa, J. (1988). *The burden of support: Young Latinos in an aging society.* Stanford: Stanford University Press.

Humm-Delgado, D. and Delgado, M. (1983). Assessing hispanic mental health needs: Issues and approaches. *Journal of Community Psychology* 11: 363-375.

Newcomb, M.B. and Bentler, P.M. (1988). *Consequences of adolescent drug use: Impact on the lives of young adults.* Newbury Park, NJ: Sage Publications.

Pinal, J.H. del and Navas, C. De (1990). *The Hispanic population in the United States: March 1989.* Washington, DC: U.S. Department of Commerce, Bureau of the Census.

Rio, A., Santisteban, D.A., and Szapocznik, J. (1990). Treatment approaches for Hispanic drug-abusing adolescents. In R. Glick and J. Moore (Eds.) *Drugs in Hispanic communities.* New Brunswick, NJ: Rutgers University Press.

Singer, M. (1984). Spiritual healing and family therapy: Common approaches to the treatment of alcoholism. *Family Therapy* 11: 152-162.

Singer, M. and Borrero, M. (1984). Indigenous treatment for alcoholism: The case of Puerto Rican spiritism. *Medical Anthropology* 8: 246-273.

Valdiveso, R. and Davis, C. (1988). *U.S. Hispanics: Challenging issues for the 1990s.* Washington, DC: Population Reference Bureau, Inc.

Valle, R. and Bensussen, G. (1985). Hispanic social networks, social support, and mental health. In W.A. Vega and M.R. Miranda (Eds.). *Stress and Hispanic mental health: Relating research to service delivery.* Rockville, MD: National Institute of Mental Health.

Valle, R. and Vega, W. (1980). *Hispanic natural support systems: Mental health promotion perspectives.* Sacramento, CA: State of California.

Index

Page numbers followed by the letter "f" indicate figures; those followed by the letter "t" indicate tables; and those followed by the letter "n" indicate notes.

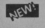
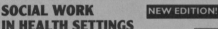

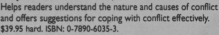

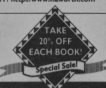